LIVING WITH DIABETES, A FAMILY AFFAIR

LIVING WITH DIABETES, A FAMILY AFFAIR
Practical and Emotional Support Strategies

by JULIE V. WATSON

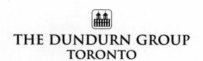

THE DUNDURN GROUP
TORONTO

Copy-Editor: Jennifer Bergeron
Design: Andrew Roberts
Printer: Transcontinental

Library and Archives Canada Cataloguing in Publication

Watson, Julie V., 1943-
   Living with diabetes, a family affair : practical and emotional support strategies / Julie V. Watson.

ISBN-10: 1-55002-551-1
ISBN-13: 978-1-55002-551-4

   1. Diabetes–Popular works.   2. Diabetics–Family relationships.   I. Title.

RC660.4.W38 2005   616.4'62   C2005-900942-X

1   2   3   4   5   09   08   07   06   05

We acknowledge the support of the Canada Council for the Arts and the Ontario Arts Council for our publishing program. We also acknowledge the financial support of the Government of Canada through the Book Publishing Industry Development Program and The Association for the Export of Canadian Books, and the Government of Ontario through the Ontario Book Publishers Tax Credit program, and the Ontario Media Development Corporation.

Printed and bound in Canada.
Printed on recycled paper.

www.dundurn.com

Dundurn Press 8 Market Street, Suite 200 Toronto, Ontario, Canada M5E 1M6	Gazelle Book Services Limited White Cross Mills Hightown, Lancaster, England LA1 4X5	Dundurn Press 2250 Military Road Tonawanda NY U.S.A. 14150

LIVING WITH DIABETES, A FAMILY AFFAIR

This book is dedicated to the members of our "team." We are so blessed to have them in our life with diabetes:

- Helen Grant, to whom I owe my sanity and well-being;
- Dr. George Carruthers, who took us on when getting a doctor was tough and is a true gem — compassionate, caring, and a darn good family physician;
- Dr. John Dornan, Endocrinology and Internal Medicine Specialist, Saint John Regional Hospital, who gave us hope and restored both health and quality of life. We especially appreciate the willingness to be flexible;
- Linda Graham, Department Manager, Diabetes Education Centre, Saint John Regional Hospital, who put us on the right track, became our lifeline, and is valued and appreciated;
- Melany Hellstern, Account Development Manager, Canada, Disetronic Medical Systems Inc., who went far beyond being simply a salesperson, helping Jack to research, understand, and become part of the wonderful world of pumping; and
- the friends who do their best to cope with the complications that we throw at them.

More than anything, this book is for Jack, who has my eternal respect, devotion, and love.

TABLE OF CONTENTS

INTRODUCTION

I never felt that I was really affected by my dad's diabetes. By the time he was really sick I had left home to go to college. I knew he was sick a lot, but looking back I realize my parents protected me from a lot of what was going on. I live in Vancouver so I would only see them during visits and it just didn't sink in. It wasn't until there was a huge improvement that I realized how sick he had been.

The biggest impact it had, the biggest thing I can think of, was when he started counting carbs and got his insulin pump. The first time I saw him after that he looked 100 percent better.

I just went, "Holy Cow! Look at you!"

I see it when we golf and do things together. He's great! We didn't do as much before, and now I realize he couldn't. I'm starting to watch my own health now. I worry that Dad was a third-generation diabetic.

— John Watson,
son of Jack and Julie Watson

One of the most difficult parts of writing a book, at least for me, is organizing it. This one is particularly difficult because there is so much I want to say — so much that needs saying. As well, it's a complex topic. I have no medical background, and neither does my husband, who is the hero of the piece. We did not intend to produce a medical book or to give medical advice.

What we wanted to do was share our story, to try to get other diabetics to take their disease seriously and work to maintain good health. We also wanted to tell the stories of other diabetics and their families with the objective of letting people know that they are not alone, they are not crazy, they are not hypochondriacs or whiners, they are not making a mountain out of a molehill, they are not seeking attention.

We felt that by reading about the experiences of others, by sharing their concerns, by using them as role models, other families could learn to cope and manage.

As importantly, we wanted to encourage people to take control. Our own experience from day one was that we had to fight and work for proper treatment and recognition of what we were dealing with and what we feel are our rights.

I had to decide early on whether I would approach doctors, the professionals, and ask them to contribute to this book. After much mind searching and discussion with others affected by the disease I decided not to do so. The reason is my own personal mandate. It always seems to me that talking to others, hearing their experiences and how they handled things first-hand, makes their stories come alive. To try to do a book that involved medical professionals would have limited my ability to tell the stories — space would have been an issue. I truly believe there is a need for a Canadian book with input from medical professionals, but this isn't it.

I didn't want it to turn into a preachy, "you must do this" book. What I want is more of a sharing, maybe a few laughs as you recognize familiar experiences, that will perhaps give all concerned a feeling of normalcy and hope that there are things they can do to maintain their quality of life. The people quoted in these pages — and there are many of them — either have diabetes or are one of the caregivers or support team for a diabetic. They are all influenced and affected by the disease.

It is important for you to know that this is not a medical book. It will not tell you how to treat your diabetes. We have no more smarts than any other layperson about this devastating disease.

What we have is the certainty that there is a gap in information out there. I get so tired of picking up magazines and specialty publications with what looks like interesting and beneficial information only to find that 90 percent of it is the same old "how to prevent diabetes," or "how to cook low-carb recipes," or "new herbal cures," or promises of cures that are still ten or twenty years in the future. There is actually very little published in mainstream publications that addresses the real issue of day-to-day living. Nothing concrete for those with diabetes.

Although I am well known as a food writer, with several cookbooks to my credit, I did not want to include recipes in this book. Frankly, it's not recipes that are needed, but rather common sense and thinking through what you are eating. Nor do we need platitudes and the same old same old. We need useful information. There has been a definite lack of useful information. To my mind, the best way to get it is to learn from others who have been there.

I guess another reason for wanting to write this book is to tell all concerned how things are from the perspective of the diabetic and those who care about them. Until you have experienced the stress, the worry, the uncertainty of what to do, until you have coped with the mood swings, the frustration of seeing someone you love deteriorating even as he refuses to do the things he needs to do, the only way you can understand is by reading or hearing the stories of others.

Be they a medical professional, coworker, family member, or even a waitress in a restaurant, I want people to be able to comprehend the concerns, the feelings, and the frustrations of diabetics so that these usually well-meaning people can at least feel compassion and at best offer viable help to improve the diabetic's quality of life.

All of that said, you can see why organizing the book was a challenge. Then one day very close to my deadline it hit me. Use our own experience and life as the guide. Break our own life with diabetes down into appropriate chapters, begin with a story from our own experiences, and include input from others and tips and hints that apply to that particular chapter. Most importantly, I felt, we should strive to keep our own voices, as well as those of others.

You will note that we have used initials only to identify people who shared their stories with us. The exceptions are a couple of instances where people wanted their names used. The reason for this is obvious. We wanted to protect people's privacy and we wanted them to be able to speak without fears of repercussions.

A FAMILY AFFAIR

You will also notice that I often refer to my husband, Jack, and myself as "we." That is because I firmly believe that diabetes is a family disease. While Jack obviously is the one who suffers from the physical and mental impact of the disease, my own life has been dramatically affected as well. I will attempt to tell both of our stories.

The logical place to start this piece is to introduce ourselves.

Jack and I met in Grade 4 in Brampton, Ontario. I was an immigrant kid, fresh off the boat from England. He took on the role of protector and became my best friend. With a year and a bit between us we went through school together. I, coming out of the English school system, had been accelerated so that we were in the same grade. We married when he was twenty-one and I was twenty and had our son, John, ten months later, and recently celebrated our fortieth anniversary.

Jack has had health problems all of his life — a variety of things, but often with the label "stress" thrown into the diagnostic mix. He always seemed to drop to the bottom fast — to get very ill very quickly. He would also pop back fast. When he was hospitalized there were often complications that were never explained away.

For the first twelve years of our marriage we lived in Brampton and Bramalea, Ontario, just outside of fast-growing Toronto. I worked for American Motors Corporation as the secretary to the director of data processing. Jack worked the night shift for Canada Post, sorting mail. We had a house in a subdivision and spent our vacations exploring Canada. A pretty normal life.

Dissatisfaction with the sameness of every day, along with the fact that our son was turning into a mall rat, led us to seek a new life. After checking out various locations across Canada we decided Prince Edward Island was home, sold everything, and in 1976 set out in search of a new life.

We purchased a couple of acres of land in the country. Jack went through an apprenticeship program to become an automotive mechanic. Eventually he got a job with Parks Canada, first as a mechanic, then in charge of roads and grounds care and maintenance.

John got to experience a richer, more basic life than Ontario suburbia, and after some angst I found my niche working in the media and eventually as a full-time freelance writer and author.

All our lives Jack has been a "doing" guy. Physically active. He loved horses. So much so that he trained as a farrier after our arrival in P.E.I. We kept horses and he loved to be out on the trails riding them. He wasn't bothered by living in a fairly remote area in the winter. The six to ten feet of snow that drifted into our driveway was just something to be moved, and cutting, blocking, and putting wood in the basement to burn in the wood stove was just something to get done. The long hours of work, the labour: he was up for all of the hard work that comes with country living, rural P.E.I. style.

In an attempt to make ends meet he had been working two jobs, putting in a forty-hour week at Parks Canada and continuing to shoe horses on the side. Eventually his health began to seriously break down.

His illness started when we lived in Riverdale on our small farm. He had no energy, to the point that at times he could hardly get out of bed. A trip to the bathroom would exhaust him. A strong, hardworking guy, he would push to keep going. Sometimes he would be full of energy, enjoying life. But those times became less and less frequent.

It was rough, especially in the winter when he would be on the road after dark. On stormy days he would leave the house at 5:00

a.m., before the plows got there to clear our rural roads. Snow was often so deep that they cancelled school and I couldn't get to work. Yet Jack would get through. At night I would stand by the window watching until he pulled in the drive.

It was a tense time. Our house was located in a perfect place for snow to drift in and fill the driveway. In the course of an hour it could ground drift as high as my waist. We had a neighbour who cleared the drive in time for me to come in from work, but Jack would often trail in several hours late. Many an evening I dug snow until I cried in frustration just so that he would not have to face it when he got home. When he did he was often so exhausted I would have to help him from his truck and up the drive to the house. Once there he would collapse into a chair and barely rouse himself to eat before dropping off to sleep. Only to do it all again the next day.

We worked valiantly to keep a social life. Often that was spending a weekend afternoon with good friends watching rented movies, keeping warm by the wood stove as winter winds blew outside. Jack just didn't have the energy for much else.

It was no way to live, for anyone. Then finally we got the diagnosis that was to change our lives forever. Jack had diabetes and needed radical change if he was to survive.

So much has happened since then. We've gone on with our lives, made adjustments, and learned to cope with what was thrown at us. We had to figure out so much on our own. We had to fight so many battles.

Things have improved vastly for diabetics today. There is education. There is much better medical treatment. There are support groups and easily accessible information sources.

Unfortunately there is no cure for diabetes yet, and when one comes it will be too late for most of the people fighting the disease today. But management tools and techniques are improving all of the time.

The seed of an idea for this book had been lurking in my head for a few years. I wanted to fill a gap in information. I just didn't feel qualified to do it. Then, one of those new tools, the insulin pump, became the water that triggered the seed to grow from a flitting idea to a determination. The first factor was our own search for information about insulin pumps. Where we lived there was virtually none at that time. We wanted to talk to people who had a pump, to find out more about them. Later, after we got an insulin pump for Jack and he experienced such a positive change in his quality of life, we wanted to share our experience with others, to spread the word about this option for treatment.

I was also increasingly aware of the need for us to become our own advocates. I found the inadequacies of the medical system in dealing with the disease to be scary, and especially the fact that where you live makes so much difference to the care and treatment you receive.

There also seemed to be a huge amount of misinformation floating around. I'm writing this as the low- / no-carb diet craze hits. It scares me how people blindly believe, and even act on, things they read. Many diabetics think some new product out there is a miraculous answer for them. Not so, folks. You need to learn to really read the labels, to think about your overall diet. There are no quick cures.

But the amount of misinformation out there is minimal when compared to the amount of non-information. I'm appalled at the number of magazines and special publications there are jumping on to the diabetes bandwagon (after all, folks, there are about sixty thousand new diabetics diagnosed in Canada each year — a huge market for the money-makers to target). Unfortunately, the majority of magazines

> **INSULIN PUMPS** are marvellous mechanical devices that replace the need for insulin injections, bringing huge benefits to diabetics. Computerized and programmable, they deliver fast-acting insulin in very small precise amounts twenty-four hours a day. Extra doses or larger amounts of insulin can be taken as needed. The pump delivers insulin via a plastic catheter to a small needle inserted through the skin. Pumps are tools operated by the diabetic to gain better control, allow more flexibility in day-to-day living, and improve overall health. For more information about insulin pumps refer to page 187.

with a flasher promoting an article on diabetes displayed on their covers are essentially promoting a food article. Many contain lots of recipes and pretty pictures. A bit thrown in about prevention ties the recipes to diabetes. Don't they realize that people interested in articles about diabetes usually have the disease already and don't need to read the same old stuff about prevention?

Oh, they often throw in a bit of news — the latest possible new "cures" that might just become reality in a decade or two, or some information about advertisers' new products. But rarely is there any truly helpful advice for those who actually have diabetes. To get that you need a specialty publication, like *Diabetes Dialogue*, the magazine published by the Canadian Diabetes Association.

Publications that are backed up by solid research and professional contributors should be a part of your ongoing education and management program. Just be careful about which you choose and look for collaborating sources before acting on anything you read, especially if it involves herbal medicines or different eating programs. Discuss those with your doctor first.

You will find no advice or instructions on how to eat, how to medicate, or how to treat your disease in this book. What we offer is general knowledge, common sense advice, and most importantly a sharing of our experiences and those of other diabetics, their supporters, and their "team" members.

One other thing. Since this is not a medical book in any way or sense we will use common language rather than medical speak. Our objective is to fill a void by sharing the stories of your peers. We will address the issue of lifestyle. This book is about facing your reality, taking charge, and working towards a good, positive life.

Two small notes before I carry on. First, although I speak about a particular drugstore, hospital, and type of insulin pump, I am not advocating them as the only choices. They are what we selected. It is up to you to research and compare.

Also, I have gone into great detail about some of our personal experiences, such as the insulin pump startup. Some will say that people today want short reads, micro bits of information. However, it has been our experience that people want detailed stories of how things worked. They want to know what is involved and how to go about it. I hope that works for you, the reader.

Jack and I have lived with diabetes for twenty years. We feel we have had an odyssey of sorts. A voyage of discovery. Our story comes from a small province where not all services are readily available. That will ensure that those of you who live in rural areas can relate. Those of you who live in cities with large populations and more medical services close by will face different challenges. I suspect a harder time getting an appointment, or even getting a doctor, will be one. In these times of government cutbacks we are all finding it harder and harder to get the medical treatment we need. I also suspect that our challenge of distance to medical services is easier to deal with than your shorter trips with denser traffic and more stressful driving conditions.

My one hope for *Living With Diabetes* is that it will give readers some encouragement to pursue what works best for both the diabetic and his or her care team.

"I feel that this book that you are researching will be a vital step in what a person in my situation has to deal with every day. I have plenty of support in how to deal with health issues and what to eat and what not to eat, how much to eat and how to regulate my blood sugars, but I do feel that there is not a whole lot of support out there for a person's day-to-day feelings on how they should deal with the hand that they have been dealt."

— MS of
New Brunswick

CHAPTER 1

Diagnosed and Moving Forward

I'm not by nature a worrier, but now I was scared. Jack was having so many strange symptoms: almost passing out, sudden fatigue, binge eating. He was also having mood swings, ranging from high to low — one day cheerful, happy, and full of energy, and another day irritable, depressed, and exhausted to the point of shuffling his feet like an old man. It had been going on for months.

All through this time we had been going to a local doctor trying to get some help with Jack's health, but we were very dissatisfied with his level of care. I started trying to diagnose Jack myself. I began recording what was happening. The erratic symptoms seemed to be related to his work schedule and, more importantly, to how he was eating. If he shoed horses after work he would not eat until he got home. Starving, he would eat a big meal and then go to bed.

I was pretty sure that his problem was related to blood sugar, but his doctor kept diagnosing "depression" and giving him tranquillizers. When I barged in one day and requested that he be sent in for a glucose tolerance test, the doctor was enraged and asked me to leave. I didn't really know what I was talking about, but my research had made that sound like a sensible thing to do. I really wanted to explore physical reasons for what was happening to Jack.

Jack himself was really not capable of arguing his case by that point. I figured he was either going to end up in a mental health facility or die if I didn't do something. If he didn't, I would. It was miserable trying to look after him, trying to keep the appearance that everything was okay for the sake of our son, working full-time and picking up the slack in the parenting part of life, and keeping up with household chores.

We had horses to feed and muck out, dogs and cats to care for, minor hockey and the joys of being twenty-five miles from town with a son in his teens not yet able to drive. We heated our home with a wood stove, meaning wood had to be brought in daily. I felt I was near the breaking point myself, when I saw an ad in the paper. A new doctor was coming to town and looking for patients. A woman.

I picked up the phone and made an appointment for myself. I was not sick, but I wanted a chance to present my case for getting Jack tested. My past experience with doctors was that they would consider only what evidence they saw on a given day. If it was a good day for the patient, then nothing appeared to be wrong. I was the hysterical wife.

I had another obstacle to contend with: Jack himself. Time after time, he would have a bad experience, I would make an appointment, and he would go to the doctor and not tell him what was happening. He would minimize it. It's a man thing. He didn't want anyone, especially his employer, to know how sick he was. I think a big part of that lies with the doctor we had at the time. He kept telling Jack it was all in his head. So Jack believed him — and there was no way he was telling the world he was crazy.

Fortunately our new doctor listened to what I was saying. She agreed to see Jack and to consider doing the testing I had suggested if she felt it was appropriate after she spoke with him. My next challenge was getting Jack to see her and tell her what was wrong. I nagged, threatened, and begged. He finally gave in. The doctor arranged for him to go into the hospital for testing, and just a few days later she called us in to tell us that, yes, Jack was diabetic.

She probably thought we were nuts when we reacted with such joy. Finally, someone was ready to acknowledge that he was very ill. That he needed proper treatment, not yet another prescription for antidepressants. Although, the treatment he got from that first doctor was enough to depress anyone!

Like most Type 2 diabetics he was treated first with diet, then with pills, but it wasn't until he went onto insulin that we really felt in control, and that was tenuous. That story will continue in later chapters.

I literally thanked God many, many times for the doctor who listened to our concerns and gave us the help we needed to manage Jack's health.

It is important for anyone reading this to remember that our experience was twenty years ago. Today the medical community is much more knowledgeable about the disease, and testing methods have improved vastly. The fact that Jack's father had diabetes and his grandfather died from the disease would prompt today's physicians to test him much earlier than it was done. I firmly believe that he would have been diagnosed quickly had he presented the same symptoms today.

Many strides have been made in the diagnosis and treatment of diabetes. Perhaps one of the most important, at least from the diabetic's perspective, is the increased amount of information available and the focus on management by the individual.

Realistically, you have to understand — at least the basics — to be in control. Control is life.

SO WHAT IS DIABETES?

The Canadian Diabetes Association says it is a lifelong condition in which your body cannot properly use and store the fuel (sugar) you take in from foods you eat.

WHAT TYPE ARE YOU?

There are basically three types of diabetes:

Type 1

Here the body either doesn't produce any insulin or not enough. Only about 10 percent of diabetics have Type 1. It is most often treated by a combination of meal planning, exercise, and daily injections of insulin. Type 1 needs good management. Before the discovery of insulin, people with Type 1 diabetes would fall into a diabetic coma and die, usually within a few weeks of onset.

Type 2

This occurs when the pancreas produces some insulin, but not enough, or when the body can't use insulin properly. Many Type 2 diabetics can control their blood sugar levels by losing excess weight, eating a healthy diet, and getting the proper amount of regular physical activity. For some, pills or insulin injections are necessary. For most, it is very important to lose weight. Extra pounds interfere with the body's ability to convert glucose to energy. The good news is that even a modest weight loss helps insulin to do a better job — and helps you to feel better. Type 2 most often occurs in people over the age of forty-five. It accounts for about 90 percent of all diabetics.

Gestational

This temporary condition occurs during pregnancy in a small percentage of women. The bad news is that it increases the risk for both mother and child of developing diabetes later on.

When you consume a meal your body converts the sugars and starches in the food to glucose, which is the fuel, or energy, your body needs. This process, turning food into energy, is sometimes called metabolism. To metabolize glucose properly, your body requires insulin, a hormone produced by the pancreas, a gland found just beneath the stomach.

The medical condition known as diabetes results from either a lack of insulin or the body's decreased ability to use insulin properly.

Insulin allows sugar, or glucose, to enter the body's cells to be converted into energy. Important stuff, insulin is also necessary for the body to make proteins and store fats. Without it, sugar and fats stay in the bloodstream. During our first education session about diabetes the instructor used a cartoon of a group of elves (insulin) catching sugar, loading it into wheelbarrows, and trundling it through the blood vessels towards an exit. That image always stayed with me. Insulin was carting away the sugar.

So, simply put, the insulin is the regulator. It prevents a build-up of sugar in the blood while ensuring that various tissues have sufficient glucose to function efficiently. When insulin isn't present to do its job, glucose levels increase dramatically in the blood and urine, causing diabetes. That presence of glucose is why diabetics do so many finger pricks. It gives a to-the-minute report of blood sugar levels, which is vital to good control.

That control is important because, over time, the presence of sugar and fat not removed by insulin damages the heart and other vital body organs. If left untreated, abnormally high levels of glucose in the blood will damage small and large blood vessels. Because the damage occurs slowly over time, we are not aware that it is contributing to heart disease, stroke, vision loss, kidney failure, nerve damage, and poor circulation in the legs and feet.

Consider this. A brochure put out by Shoppers Drug Mart, titled "Diabetes," says:

> Diabetes is a chronic disease that has no cure, but it can be managed. Education is the key to controlling diabetes, but experts estimate that 30% of people with Type 1 diabetes and 70% of those with Type 2 never receive appropriate education about diabetes and self-care. About 40% of people with diabetes will develop complications at some point, but early diagnosis and close management can help prevent or delay complications that can have serious health consequences.

Those complications can include high blood pressure, heart disease, stroke, high cholesterol, eye disease, kidney disease, nerve damage, foot problems, liver and pancreatic cancer, and something that the "experts" tend to ignore: mood swings, irritability, and depression.

TREATMENTS AND MEDICATIONS

Basically there are two types of medication used to help control blood sugar levels. Your doctor will determine which, if any, you need.

The first is insulin, which is a hormone, not a medicine. It replaces the insulin that your own pancreas should be producing. Insulin is prescribed for Type 1 diabetes and sometimes for Type 2. There are several types of insulin, which we layfolk basically distinguish as quick-acting, short-acting, long-acting, or a mixture.

PHARMACISTS such as those found at Shoppers Drug Mart can be very valuable tools in your health care plan. Pharmacists not only supply you with drugs, they are also very knowledgeable about how various drugs interact, about tools and supplies such as log books available to you, and more. They usually have information available free of charge. One of the benefits of the information prepared by national chains and distributed through their pharmacies is its readability. Most of it is very easy to understand, and the pharmacists can answer most questions you will have.

Then there are pills, glucose-lowering medicines that are sometimes prescribed for Type 2 diabetics. Again there are several different drugs that do the job, all with different characteristics.

Sometimes it takes experimentation and adjustment to get the treatment that works best for you. You and your doctor must work together, keeping track of your sugars and how you feel.

Your doctor also has to balance what you are taking for your diabetes with other drugs that may be prescribed to you. You must be aware that some drugs, both prescription and non-prescription, should not be taken by diabetics. You must tell your doctor about everything that you are taking, even vitamins and herbal supplements.

Beware of cough and cold remedies; buy only sugar-free and alcohol-free products. You should always check with a pharmacist and read the labels on products carefully. Pay attention to the cautions and warnings.

CONTROL — A VITAL INGREDIENT FOR HEALTH

Now you know why control is vital.

When you are diagnosed as a diabetic you have some important decisions to make. Are you going to bury your head in the sand, or are you going to step up, learn what you need to learn, act on it, and improve your quality of life?

Are you going to do everything you can for yourself and for those who love and care about you, or are you going to pretend the disease doesn't exist and subject yourself and those same people to a future that can include some nasty medical realities, a lesser quality of life, and even death?

> ### MEDICATION BALANCING ACT
>
> There is a reason diabetics have to be careful with medications. Mistakes can make you sick. You must pay attention to what you are doing. Low blood sugar (a.k.a. hypoglycemia, insulin reaction, or insulin shock) can be caused by taking too much medication, eating too little food, or exercising too much.

The decisions diabetics make — to work for their own well-being or to passively submit to the disease — will affect the future lives of both themselves and who care about them or are dependent on them for their own happiness.

Sounds harsh. And it is. A diagnosis of diabetes is a reality check. Is that piece of pie, that late meal, that high-sugar beverage so important to you that you are willing to sacrifice your vision, your ability to play ball with your children, to make love to your wife, to continue in your job, to go on vacations, to simply feel good?

So here you are, diagnosed with diabetes and hopefully determined to manage it to the best of your ability. You've been to the doctor and have your treatment program. Perhaps you have an eating plan to follow. You should also have the information needed to get yourself to some education sessions or training. It is absolutely vital that you follow through. Go to the classes; learn as much as you can. For when it comes to diabetes, knowledge combined with appropriate action truly is power.

If you are having trouble accepting that you must now manage what you eat, when you eat, how much exercise you get in a day, medications, and so on, sit down in a quiet place and ask yourself a few simple questions:

- What do I want out of life?
- What things do I want to do?
- What do I want to see?
- Do I want to enjoy my children's future — see them graduate, get married, achieve their dreams?
- Do I want to share Thanksgiving and Christmas dinner with my grandchildren?
- Do I want to play golf, walk that nature trail, ride that motorcycle?
- Where would I like to go for a vacation? Can I go there?
- What do I want to do in my retirement?
- What am I willing to give up?
- Would I willingly hurt my wife, my children, my siblings, my friends?

Think about the rest of your life and what you want from it. We all face health concerns and medical problems as we age, but we can minimize them, delay them, and reduce their impact on our lives. One of the questions diabetics should consider is this: do I want those things in my life sooner or later?

Now ask yourself two final questions. Can I do all of these things if I am sick? Am I willing to close the door on my dreams because I'm too lazy, too stubborn, too weak to make some changes?

If you do not have a referral for education sessions call the nearest branch of the Canadian Diabetes Association. Its first mandate is to educate the public about diabetes. I also suggest joinng the Canadian Diabetes Association to obtain its publications, such as *Diabetes Dialogue*, a helpful magazine. If there isn't a local branch office near you, call 1-800-BANTING, email info@diabetes.ca, or go to the association's website at http://www.diabetes.ca.

It is important to note that the level and quality of services available may not be the same at all branches across the country. If you don't feel satisfied at your local branch, rest assured that the information from the national office is the same all across the country and join it, instead. That's what I did.

After being diagnosed with diabetes, it is very important that you learn everything you can about how to live with and treat the disease. Here in Canada we are fortunate in having good information available through various diabetic education centres.

DGA (remember, we are using initials to protect privacy) of Prince Edward Island can't say enough about the importance of attending education sessions and her good opinion of the staff who present the programs. She also stresses the importance of having someone go with you, because there is so much information that it can be overwhelming.

JG and her daughter, DGA, are an example of how things should be handled after a senior is diagnosed with diabetes. Actually, let me revise that. It should read how *everyone* should handle those initial days. There is a lot to learn and absorb. Having a spouse, relative, or friend with you at the education sessions helps you to remember and makes it easier to get into this new way of living.

What was DGA's reaction when her mother was diagnosed? "Oh good grief, what next? Mom has had to cope with many things in her life: rheumatic fever, Bell's palsy, breast cancer — twice — tremors in legs, weakness, all that sort of stuff."

SENIOR MOM AND ADULT DAUGHTER TEAM UP

JG is a senior with some mobility and health problems who lives alone in an apartment. DGA, her daughter, lives several miles away with her husband. She works from home. I asked her if there is any way her mother would have, or could have, taken in everything that was presented during their sessions at the Diabetes Education Centre and remembered it.

"I look at the pages of notes I took, two, three, four pages each session," she says. "I know Mom is not capable of taking all of that in and retaining it. She has a hearing problem so wouldn't have heard it all. For me, writing it down jogs your memory. It helps you remember."

DGA is the type of person who gets a lot out of any education session she attends because of the way she approaches it. "If I have a question, I ask. Lots of times there are so many things to remember it's hard for anyone, so writing down what the teacher is saying, having notes, helps."

It also helped her to confirm or restate things with her mother.

"One thing was re-calibrating her test meter. She remembered that she has to do calibrating, but didn't remember you have to do it for each vial. There are two per box. She hadn't remembered that you have to do it for each container, not each box."

When her mom experienced some unusual readings, being able to check back in the notes helped this mother/daughter team to keep on track and eliminated the potential for arguments.

DGA deserves a lot of credit not only for spending the time to make sure her mom got to her sessions but also for staying with her, learning with her, and becoming an important part of her management team. She's proud of her mom, who has not only been widowed in recent years but also had numerous health challenges.

Part of the reason JG is doing so well is the dedication of her daughter. When they obtained her monitor for testing blood sugars they got a free instruction video. DGA watched it twice herself, then took it to her mom's and watched it with her. They then watched it two more times, doing it with the meter until JG was confident doing it on her own.

"I'm so amazed and proud of how well she is doing. Practically had to force her to eat a piece of her own birthday cake. I just wish my sisters and brothers also went to the sessions. I try to tell them, but...."

She has nothing but praise for the training they received. "I did a lot of preaching about the Diabetes Education Centre after she was done. Mother just doesn't tune in to all this stuff. I got her a MedicAlert bracelet and Lifeline. They were great with information about what to do, how to do it, and patient."

In describing her mother, DGA says that she gets a notion in her head and she's gonna do it. "I'm so thankful that she was open to going to the Diabetes Education Centre. Her only negative comment was 'It's a lot of running around, isn't it.'

"I can't say enough about how wonderful the staff was in there. It's too bad you have to have a relative or friend with diabetes to go to the sessions. I was better informed than most through friends having it [diabetes], but I was still amazed at what I didn't know."

DGA strongly urges diabetics and those who support them in managing their disease to seek out and attend diabetes education sessions with the determination to learn how to manage the disease properly. "Take someone with you to take notes and go over things with you later. It's a lot of information."

"One of the most off-putting things for newly diagnosed diabetics is the thought of needles, of pricking your finger with a needle to do testing, and of giving injections. Like everything, once the initial fear is overcome, you can do it. This is where people will get over those fears.

"For instance, they had a lot of information about testing and testers [at the education sessions]. Mother wanted to look at the arm-testing thing, but I pointed out that you still have to prick yourself. She resisted the idea, but we stressed the need to get blood and that the only way to do it is to prick yourself so that you bleed. So she just started testing."

With the support of the people at the Diabetes Education Centre and a supportive, patient daughter, JG has licked that fear and now confidently tests according to the schedule set out for her.

As upsetting as it is to have a parent, an older person, diagnosed with diabetes, I can only imagine the reaction of a parent being told his or her beloved child has the disease. DOH of Ontario gives us some insight.

YOUNG DAUGHTER AND HER MOM LEARN TO COPE

DOH's daughter, twelve years old at the time of writing, has Type 1 diabetes and is insulin dependent. She was diagnosed when she was six years old. "She requires insulin injections [between three and six a day] for the rest of her life unless a cure is found. Since diagnosed, she has received close to seven thousand injections. That's a lot of hurt. Plus she must test her blood sugars at least four times a day, which requires her to poke blood from her fingertips. She must also match her insulin intake to the amount of carbohydrates she eats, as well as take into consideration the amount of exercise and stress she has, what the weather is like outside [because insulin works differently in cold versus hot weather], and whether she has a cold or has eaten simple or complex carbohydrates. It's not a simple science."

The diagnosis of diabetes was not an easy one for the family to hear.

"Initially diabetes knocked the wind from our family's sail. We had a tight knit family but slowly each one of us started to unravel until the whole family structure not only looked frayed but appeared beyond repair. Emotions swung from denial to rage to guilt to tears to depression. We felt trapped when our freedom was lost. We needed to follow a strict schedule of eating certain amounts of food at certain times of day, in order to match the type of insulin that was given. We worried about whether we had given too much or not enough insulin and naturally we wondered about the future, whether diabetes would shorten the life expectancy of our child or cause her to suffer with eye, kidney, or heart damage.

"Most families that we've met feel isolated from the general public. It's frightening to talk about the stories which we share amongst ourselves only because the general public has no clue, nor do they want to know or understand what it's like. It's too painful.

"And yet, despite the negative feelings, a time comes when the tables turn and the family picks up all the loose ends and finds a new strength. Today, our lives feel relatively normal. The fear is still there and every once in awhile a situation crops up that reminds us of how much we hate diabetes.

"Still, because of the diabetes, we have met some great people, done things we would have never done, followed dreams that were sitting in a drawer, and came to realize that the most important thing in life is family and the love of people. We live in a material world but I see so much money being wasted on such frivolous items. Money is needed for research, not another dress in one's closet."

The diagnosis brought many frustrations and responsibilities to the family, along with the personal impact on everyday life. This mom quickly realized that the battle is far more reaching.

"A family living with diabetes faces many challenges. Initially, there is so much to learn. I don't know how some families cope.

Today, the real challenge is finding a cure and encouraging people that additional research can make a difference. Everyone has a role to play, but life itself is so hectic that people can't seem to find the time to do the little extras anymore. I'm in the same boat as everyone else. More time, more research dollars, and more education. That's what is needed."

As a parent she always feels responsible for keeping her child healthy, and in this role DOH has taken great steps to understand, to educate herself, and to work for her daughter and the diabetic community.

"She is my daughter, my only child. Now that she is twelve she is finally doing her own insulin injections at school. Prior to that I needed to hang around home, planning my outings around her schedule. Eventually the responsibility will all be passed to my daughter, but in the meantime, our whole family shares in the workload. My husband especially is a great help and he is deeply missed when he's out of town or working late or on weekends.

"The timing of injections and meals used to be a concern, but as you learn more about diabetes and become more comfortable in the care, you learn to break the rules, which allows more flexibility in the timing of meals and injections. The introduction of insulin pumps as well as fast-acting insulins such as NovoRapid and Humalog were instrumental in returning some freedom back to the person with diabetes. It is getting easier and we are thankful we are dealing with this condition now versus pre-insulin days when the diagnosis of diabetes was a death sentence. Insulin controls the situation but it is *not* a cure," she stresses.

"Everyone learns to deal with diabetes in their own way. I've learned there is no magic formula. For the longest time, my daughter was in denial, which in the short term made caring for her diabetes less stressful than when she was upset. However, eventually the feelings must surface, and when they did, the emotions were intensified tenfold.

"My husband buried himself in his work. Like my daughter, he didn't want to talk about it. The sooner he returned to his normal routine, the better.

"For me, finding close friends in a local support group prepared me for the worst. I needed to read, learn as much as I could about diabetes and become an expert. Allow yourself to control the diabetes rather than have it control you. Becoming involved as a volunteer with the local branch of the Canadian Diabetes Association also helped. However, the best advice came from another mother who was also coping with a child with diabetes. She said to find three passions and to follow at least one of them each day. Whenever I just couldn't cope any more I buried myself in my gardening, writing, and reading. It worked."

TESTING YOUR BLOOD — THE KEY TO CONTROL

Probably the most important thing that anyone with diabetes must do for themselves is maintain careful control of blood sugar levels. How often you do it depends on the type of diabetes you have. But, no matter the type, all diabetics should test their blood sugar regularly. And it should be done with a good blood glucose monitor. We call 'em testers. There are dozens on the market, and many of them have gone through our house in the past few years.

OUCH!

Many people associate testing their blood, which requires pricking their finger, with pain. It does get easier as your fingers get toughened. And here is a tip: don't prick the sensitive tip, the middle of your fingerprint where all the swirls are. There are all kinds of nerve endings there, and you use the tips of your fingers all of time, irritating them if they are sore. Instead prick to the sides of your finger pad. You can also explore the new testers that can be used to sample from your arm.

Basically you must prick your finger and squeeze a small sample of blood onto a special area on the end of a test strip. The machine then "reads" the blood and tells you your blood sugar level at that moment in time. Cool, huh! You instantly know whether you are high, low, or in control. This easy testing is a major development in diabetes management.

It is important to test at times or in circumstances determined with your management team. You should follow a schedule and record the results of your test properly. These test results are the tool that your doctor or educator will use to adjust your food intake, physical activity, and medication. All the better to control your diabetes.

Checks show how activities affect your blood sugars. Jack, for instance, is an avid golfer. He checks his sugars around the ninth hole.

If you want to try out several different testers, head for your local Canadian Diabetes Association office. They often have several different ones on hand. Or ask your pharmacist; the pharmacy might have a demo day or be willing to show you various models. Testers, like all gadgets, are becoming more and more sophisticated. Personally, I think it's important to get one that you feel happy with. Go too high tech and you might find it difficult to master. Make sure that you can read the screen.

Important things to consider when choosing a tester are ease of use, being able to read the results easily, the cost of strips, the size (you have to carry it around with you), the speed, and the availability of supplies. This is very important if you travel, in which case you should purchase from a national chain of pharmacies.

Price is also a consideration, but there are often great deals on obtaining testers at your pharmacy. The manufacturers want you to buy their test strips — this is where the profit is — so the tester (or monitor) is often available free or at low cost. Considering the fact that your tester is probably your most important management tool, it is very important that you choose one that works for you.

After you get a tester, send in the paperwork that comes with it. Once the manufacturers have you on their mailing list you will receive special offers, free samples, and so on that help cut the costs a little and keep you up to date on new developments.

These days Jack uses a tester that has the strips preloaded into a cartridge. He pushes the button and the strip pops out, ready for a wee tiny drop of blood. It's fast and he basically likes it. It does spoil the occasional strip, so that adds to the costs of operation.

The cost is important to consider. Some strips cost about a dollar apiece. Jack tests four to eight times a day depending on what he is doing, how he feels, and whether he is charting for his doctor. Strips are a major cost for us. He also opted for a tester that holds a number of strips in a drop-in cartridge, rather than having to open a little foil packet each time and insert the test strip in the meter. He made the move to this Accu-Chek tester when his eyesight was bad, and also because he tests so much it is often done in the car, when we are out walking, in a restaurant, or wherever he happens to be.

Many diabetics don't need to test that often. Just remember that the tester shows you where your blood sugars are at that moment. It shows you how well you are controlling your diabetes.

If a diabetic is feeling "off" or poorly, if he feels out of whack, like his sugars are high or low, the first thing he should do is test. Testing lets you know whether this is a blood sugar problem or something else, such as the flu, a cold, something you ate, or something you need to talk to your doctor about.

A good friend of ours recently presented me with a what-not-to-do example when we went out to lunch. He regulates his diabetes with pills and diet. A group of us were just giving our orders to the waitress when he said he was feeling bad. His wife asked the waitress to bring an order of french fries "in a hurry." Jack immediately asked him if his sugars were low. He didn't know. He didn't have a tester with him. But he *felt* like they were low. Jack had tested before we entered the restaurant so he offered to go to the car and get his tester. The offer was turned down, with a "No, I'll be okay."

When the french fries came he dug in, sharing with his wife. He then ate his lunch. After the meal he still didn't feel well so he went home to lie down. He slept the afternoon away.

Jack and I were flabbergasted. Because Jack is a brittle diabetic control is very important to us, so we were appalled by our friend's behaviour. When you care about someone and see him doing something that is damaging to his health you just want to yell at him or shake some sense into him. Yet you can't. We do try to point out the errors, to relate how things should be done, but when things get tense we have to back off.

So what was wrong here? First, our friend only guessed he was low. He didn't test. Unless he tested he really couldn't know; he could just as easily have been high. Second, they ordered a high-fat, slow-to-break-down plate of french fries. If he was low he needed something fast-acting, like juice or a sports drink. Finally, by eating the fries, then his full lunch, he had a very high-carb, high-fat lunch. Not something he needs with the pounds he is packing. If his sugars were high he just compounded the problem.

> Blood glucose monitors, or testers, are often referred to as **BGMs**.

Considering this couple's refusal to educate themselves about diabetes and to manage properly, I would not be surprised to learn that he is having more problems and needs to go on insulin. Being good friends with the couple, we see this ongoing behaviour often and worry about him.

TIME BUILDS UNDERSTANDING

MS of New Brunswick pointed out the importance of time when it comes to adjusting to this new way of life. She has a very valid point, one that takes us back to that basic rule, "take it one step at a time."

"I just wanted to share a small note about a conversation I had with a dietician that I live next door to. She deals with a lot of people who have to change their eating habits because they just found out that they have this disease. I told her to try and take it slow with them.

"The reason I think that a lot of people find it so difficult is that the doctors and others try to make a person change overnight. They throw too much information at a person all at once. You go to a clinic for a couple of days and are expected to take *all* this new information and change immediately. I proposed to her to try and work on one meal a day at the beginning and then eventually get all the meals worked in there to what they are supposed to be doing. She [tried my suggestion and] said that there was a remarkable improvement in people accepting the change they had to make because it came at a speed that was easier to understand."

All diabetics should do the following to protect themselves:

1. Wear a MedicAlert or similar bracelet or necklace that identifies you as a diabetic.
2. Carry a medical ID card. You can buy them or make them yourself on your computer. Or, if you don't have a computer, have a friend do one for you and get several printed: one for your wallet, others for your fanny pack, medical kit, suitcase, etc. List the following information:

   - your name, address, telephone number
   - names and phone numbers of people to contact in case of emergency
   - your physician, with address and phone number
   - medical conditions
   - allergies
   - current medications and dosages

TO GO PUBLIC — OR NOT

Many individuals are faced with a real dilemma when diagnosed with diabetes. Do I go public or not? It can be a difficult decision.

Some perceive the disease as something to be ashamed of, that it takes away from their manhood or femininity. They might fear it will jeopardize their job, cause them to lose out on promotion, or even bring a risk of being let go. Some see it as a personal stigma, while others don't want pity, and some just don't want to deal with it.

Many of those concerns are justified. But my concern is that by denying it publicly, you may be refusing to accept that you have the disease. If you don't accept that you have it, you are not going to properly manage it.

So get over it, people. Admit that this is now part of your life. There is no shame in having diabetes. It just is. You won't be pitied unless you do things that are detrimental to your health. People pity those who are doing stupid things or acting the idiot. They feel sympathy and concern for those who are doing everything they can for themselves.

As for not wanting to deal with it — you must. If you don't, you *will* get sicker, you *will* suffer from complications. Every time you are faced with something you don't want to deal with, think about it. How long will it take? How hard is it, really? Testing, for instance, takes what, a minute? Is eating on time really that bad? Is it really so awful to eat healthy? Compared to the consequences, dealing with your diabetes when and how you should is nothing more than a series of trivial things.

The one real concern here is the impact on your career or job. We address that in chapter four.

BUILD YOUR TEAM

It is very important that diabetics pay attention to acquiring a team to help and support them in developing and maintaining their management and treatment plan. Your team will probably never sit in one room for a brainstorming session, or even talk to each other about your care — unfortunately.

It is a sad fact that where you live will influence whom you can bring into your team, but this group is critical, so put work into attaining the support you need and deserve. Your list should include the following:

- a diabetic specialist
- your family physician
- specialists in health complications
- a pharmacist
- a diabetes educator
- a dietician
- your spouse or caregiver
- friends and co-workers

DEVELOP YOUR MANAGEMENT PLAN

It is a simple reality that you can't follow a plan if you don't have one. You have to know what you are supposed to do and how to do it. You have to work out a realistic plan that you can live with. Your plan must include:

- A diet designed for you. Not a general eating plan, but *your* eating requirements set out in a way that works for your life;
- An exercise program with some realistic goals. Don't set yourself up to fail by setting unrealistic goals;
- A schedule for testing and recording your results;
- A plan for taking medicine or injecting insulin properly. This should take into account your diet, exercise, and work schedule;
- A plan to quit smoking and reduce exposure to second-hand smoke.

Being diagnosed with diabetes can be one of the best moments if you have been struggling with poor health and no seeming solution for feeling better. Finally there is a name for what you are experiencing, things that can be done to counteract the symptoms, a known enemy to fight. Coping with the euphoria, thinking you are in control, getting overconfident, and ignoring lesser symptoms are normal reactions. In fact control is hard to maintain, and it is difficult to prevent sliding back into old bad habits. Hearing how others handle this phase is the best way to be alert for the best ways to care for yourself, which is why personal experience is so much a part of this book.

Advice I can't share often enough is the importance of educating yourself. One way to do that is to join the Canadian Diabetes Association so that you receive its publication *Diabetic Dialogue*. Also, do check out its website, http://www.diabetes.ca.

Another must is to attend education sessions put on by your medical community or local association. Ask your doctor to refer you or recommend some to you.

If you have been diagnosed with diabetes early, count your blessings. You have time to take control, time to drop weight and get your health on track. You won't be like GB, who said, "My step-father-in-law got diabetes. His eyes went. That's how we found out. He was never diagnosed before that. He didn't last long. He's dead now."

CHAPTER 2
Impact on Life

It's really hard to write something short about the effects diabetes has had on Jack. In the beginning the biggest impact
was the adjustments it took to try to eat meals at regular
times. Working two jobs, having varied physical activity at those
jobs that he could not predict from day to day, long hours, and
an irregular schedule that made regular meals difficult were
real challenges.

He felt much better and was able to function well as long
as he stayed in control of his routine, particularly in terms of
mealtimes. In those early days the biggest impact was social.
For years we had enjoyed a circle of friends we did fun things
with and enjoyed having in our lives. There was one couple in
particular who shared our love of horses and had sons the
same age as ours, and we got along very well. One of the things
we used to enjoy was going out for Sunday breakfast. Just us
adults. Before Jack was diagnosed that breakfast would be
between ten-thirty and eleven o'clock. When he was diagnosed
his meal plan was set around his job schedule. He had to be at
work by eight o'clock in the morning, after a drive of a half-
hour in summer and as much as an hour in winter. He ate breakfast between six o'clock and six-thirty. For him to suddenly

change his routine on a Sunday just didn't work. We tried breakfast at eight-thirty, but they hated getting up that early on their day off. We tried switching to lunch, but they weren't ready until long past his scheduled mealtime. We tried just having coffee while they ate breakfast, but they were very vocal about us making too big a deal. A couple of hours wouldn't hurt, they said.

I can't count the number of times we've heard those words, "Just this time won't matter," and from many different people.

Jack struggled to adjust to our friends. But he began to have low blood sugar reactions to the point that I would have to take over and get sugar into him far too often. He got all out of whack. Stubborn, he struggled to keep up to others' expectations, but it had a real adverse effect on his health.

In the long run he couldn't keep it up. Sunday with our friends usually left him ill. When he started having to phone in sick on Monday mornings and miss a day's work, we had to start saying no to breakfast out, losing an enjoyable part of our life.

Our relationship had to change with another set of friends. They have a farm and a routine set around working outside in daylight hours. Meals were seldom at the times Jack needed, although they were much more sensitive to his needs. Another factor was the amount of sugar she used in her cooking. Sugar in soup, in salad dressings — it all mounted up. Rather than sitting at the table saying "I can't eat that," it became easier to just not be there long enough to have a meal.

In this case the sugar was hidden. Our friend was aware Jack could not have sugar, but she wouldn't accept that molasses, for instance, is sugar. Or she would say it's only a little bit so it doesn't matter. She did eventually begin putting out things like sliced tomatoes or cucumber without the usual sprinkle of sugar, but her feelings would be hurt when Jack would not be able to eat something. He always tests before a meal and eats accordingly. He didn't feel comfortable saying no. We still count them as best friends. With our busy schedules getting together is a challenge, but what works best is the occasional meal out where he can order what works on a given day at a given time.

Which brings us to eating out in the evenings. Normally Jack ate dinner between five-thirty and six o'clock. Any later and he was in trouble. If you go out for an evening meal or special function dinner is normally served at seven-thirty or eight o'clock. Too late for us. So we seldom go.

Jack and I are members of a motorcycle touring club that organizes an annual rally in Prince Edward Island. One of the highlights of the event is the hip of beef barbecue. For several years we had to watch everyone else enjoy the meal because it was served too late in the day for Jack. Since there is no other food service at the event we had to either take sandwiches or leave the campgrounds to buy food at his scheduled eating time.

We had been social animals who shared many good times with friends that were based around eating. But when he was diagnosed with diabetes and became determined to be in control, things changed.

When we received an invitation out my first question would always have to be, "What time are you eating?" The next question was "What are you serving?" Not too difficult with friends, but when it was people who were not used to us and our routine I had to explain about Jack's diabetes and his need to stay on schedule and to know what he was eating.

Most people immediately say they will eat on time. But then the meal would be one, two, or even three hours late. Especially at holidays. I have been known to barge into a kitchen, make up a plate of food, and take it to Jack. He hated it when I did that. I have also been known to say, "Sorry, we have to leave. Jack needs to eat so we are going to a restaurant." Made me popular. We became reluctant to accept invitations out, especially from people we didn't know, and frankly people stopped inviting us.

Our answer was to invite people to our house. Socially this kept us in touch with friends. Unfortunately we began to feel slighted by people who never extended an invitation in return in a manner that Jack could enjoy and stay healthy.

Social eating caused us much pain. We felt abandoned and unimportant. We became, to a large degree, solitary creatures. It probably affected me more than it did Jack. He just adjusted and set up activities that he could enjoy with his buddies: golf, going to a hockey game. I've had a harder time letting the hurt go. It still bothers me. One particular couple ate at our home many times without ever inviting us to theirs. We still got together but on a different basis, over coffee or at a club meeting. Invariably they talk about friends they had over, the fun card games, the barbecues. Sadly, it changed relationships.

Now I might sound like a whiner, but we are talking about impact on life here. Friends, socializing, participating in activities with others are the essence of enjoying life. I think this is where a lot of diabetics fall down in their management plan, so it is something to be aware of. Jack and I realized we had to change. We had to become self-protective and put his health first. We talked about it and decided we are great as a twosome, so we don't sweat it much anymore. We still have close friends, but the dynamics have been adjusted.

As I say to people over and over again, diabetes is not a dis ease of one person — it draws the spouse or significant other as well as family and friends into its clutches. If you don't deal with it together the biggest impact can be a breakdown within your extended family unit.

That said, the other major impact is obviously on health. As you can see from the personal stories we tell at the beginning of each chapter, health and lifestyle are big issues in our own experience.

Today Jack is living an active life, but he also contends with pain and discomfort. I see him holding his back in the area of his kidneys. I see him rubbing his chest to try to ease recurring chest pain. He is often cold and gets a lot of leg pain. He doesn't shake colds, flu, or being over-tired easily. He doesn't heal as well as he used to.

He constantly manages — he counts everything he eats, he ensures he gets his daily exercise, he finger pricks and tests his blood at least five times a day. He changes the site for his insulin pump every three days religiously and ensures that he keeps the site clean. He is very careful about taking his drugs on time. He sees his specialists and physician regularly. It is time-consuming, but he does it. He follows a diet and takes supplements we have designed not only to keep him healthy but also to do the best we can for his eyes. There is never a day of freedom from the routine.

Perhaps the worst thing for him is his eyes. Jack has an ongoing relationship with his eye specialist. He has had too many laser treatments to count, lens transplants, and the stress of ongoing bad news. He has lost driving privileges, then gained them back. He is always aware of his eyes. His chair in the living room is placed so that he can see the television and, with a turn of the head, down the street. Those are his monitors. "I can't see as well today," he'll say in the morning.

We have noticed that his eyesight is tied to how he feels, how his sugars are on a particular day. We have learned that exercise affects his vision. As long as he gets exercise his vision stays stable. If he is down sick for a while, his vision is affected. Oh, he can still see, and most days see well, but there is always that awareness.

For years we planned a retirement that allowed us to travel. Now he wonders if he will be able to see enough to enjoy it. We've found that flying is too hard on him. If he can't drive or see the scenery, will he want to travel?

Also, our medical costs are constantly rising. That fact alone is changing how we envision living our senior years. One of the stresses that affect us the most is that we see his health deteriorating and would like to do some of the things we have dreamed of while he can. Instead he stresses about how we will survive financially. Living with diabetes is a very expensive lifestyle.

Jack has had to shelve some of his dreams. He has always wanted to ride across Canada on his motorcycle. This past summer he had to sell it. Not an easy decision — to give up your dream. We would love to be able to buy him a new lower rider — easier to ride — so that he could take his trip, but with the high medical costs it isn't likely to happen. Not unless we win the lottery.

Diabetes means change. Timing, measuring, and controlling become the constants that rule life. It isn't always easy. What if the kids' hockey game runs through suppertime? What if your sugar levels are all out of whack and you know you shouldn't drive? What if the family wants pizza or ice cream while they watch a movie?

Diabetics need to think these things through. Can another parent take the kids to those suppertime games? Can you take your meal with you and eat while you watch them play?

If you shouldn't drive, can your spouse, child, or friends do it? Should you call a taxi? Or can you take some sugar, wait an hour, and then drive?

Can you get a special treat for yourself on movie night so that you don't feels so bad about missing pizza or ice cream?

It all takes some thinking as you look for viable alternatives. Do a reality check. Are any of these things so important that you should risk your health or the safety of others who are in a car with you?

Yes, there is an impact on your life, as we will explore through the chapter. The good news is that you have the power to take control. To do that you need to stay healthy.

KEEPING THE "HO HO" IN HOLIDAYS

I want to talk now about what I feel is one of the most difficult times for diabetics and perhaps worse for their families. I grew up addicted to the joys of Christmas. Perhaps it's my English heritage that is responsible for my love of Christmas carols and the whole gifts under the tree, holly and ivy scenario. In my family Christmas was a time to get together, which intensified in importance after we all immigrated to Canada. Wrapping our gifts, finding our stockings, opening our presents, Christmas dinner, and our Boxing Day get-togethers with the grandparents, aunties and uncles, and cousins were all a very important part of my growing up.

The tradition continued after we were married, even after we moved to Prince Edward Island. Diabetes brought much of the enjoyment to a screeching halt. No, that's wrong. It wasn't a screeching halt; it was a slow, grinding, scraping away.

Consider these two examples from our life.

First, we have gone to visit family, people who love to party with friends and look forward to spending Christmas Eve meeting some of their dearest. This was at the time when Jack was trying to control his diabetes with diet and pills. I warned our hosts that he had to eat his meals on time and that he needed to have some basic, plain food rather than rich sauces or things that were high in sugar.

We offered to get our own meal before going out, but they were shocked that we would suggest such a thing and assured us that they would be eating on time. Of course everyone knows what happened. Jack's time to eat came and went. But we didn't. We hadn't left the house yet! Just as I had decided enough was enough and headed for the kitchen everyone headed for the car. It was a half-hour drive to the party, but we were assured we would eat as soon as we arrived. Of course we didn't, and all that was available was the usual nuts and chips. Jack was showing all the signs of low blood sugar, including irritability. He was now digging in his heels, saying he didn't need to eat.

Finally, even though our hosts were strangers, I knew I had to raid the kitchen. They were all gathered around the island drinking wine and beer, having a grand time and enjoying the slow process of making a barbecue on their indoor firepit. I was assured it would be only another couple of minutes.

Jack was slumped in a chair, but I saw him get up and head for the door. I got firm and demanded that they let me make a sand-wich *right now*. As I spoke I raided the fridge, taking some regular pop along with some food. I found him sitting in the car, almost unconscious. It was hard getting the pop and some food into him. It was hard sitting out in the cold trying to bring him around. It was harder being told I was a party pooper when we finally could go back inside. It was even harder to be stuck with a husband who needed to be able to relax and recover while we were teased and given a hard time about not joining in and spoiling other people's fun. The most difficult part of the evening was not having our own car so that we could leave.

Before we went to bed in the wee hours of the morning I again stressed that Jack must eat on time, especially after his experience that night. I woke up the next day with a feeling of dread and a knot in my stomach. It was Christmas Day, and I knew it would not go well. After present-opening I did all of the preparation for dinner while our hosts went for a nap. Jack and I had breakfast and lunch on time. When I went to start the meal cooking for serving at six o'clock I was told in no uncertain terms that the company would not be arriving until seven. Thus, dinner would not be served until eight. Jack and I had a sandwich.

We learned several things that Christmas. The first was that as a couple we had to put his needs first. Now we always go in our own car, and we just get our meal when we need to. If the people we are visiting don't care enough about us to adjust, then we do our own thing.

Another Christmas we drove many hours to be with family. When we arrived, on Christmas Eve, there was literally no food where we were staying — our brother-in-law existed by eating out or going to his girlfriend's. So our Christmas Eve supper was at the local Dairy Queen — the only place open. We bought a little stash at a convenience store for breakfast. Now we go prepared to look after ourselves, arriving with groceries.

The timing of meals over a holiday like Christmas can be a major factor for diabetics. It isn't just that we have to get our own meals. That isn't a problem; we're used to it. It's the emotional hit. It hurts when friends and family won't make a small adjustment to scheduling to include the diabetic in the celebrations. It turns what should be a day of joy into a day of stress and worry for the wife or parent of the diabetic. It makes the diabetic sick and is cruel and demeaning.

We used to always travel to family for the yule season, but we stopped. Now we stay home, reduce the stress to his body and emotions, and quietly pass the day. For me the joy of the season has been tempered. Friends try to fill the gap, and one couple in particular, Beth and David Smith, have done their best to adjust to Jack's schedule. They will never know how much that means to us.

Our Christmas experiences are a little easier now that Jack is on an insulin pump, but we still treat holidays with caution and care for his schedule.

Staying on time is difficult on this day, with the excitement of presents being opened and the arrivals and departures of friends and family. Whether you are hosting diabetics, have them in your immediate family, or are being entertained by a diabetic, please remember that the joy of the day is best preserved by the simple acts of paying attention to the clock and offering a few dishes that fit their diet. Your attention to these small things, for any holiday or special occasion, is the best demonstration of love and caring that you can give.

LIVING WITH YOUR PLAN

One of the biggest impacts on the diabetic's life is the need to live with a management plan. You need to take charge of things that many of you have never thought about before. Things like:

- setting goals that will help you take care of yourself
- planning meals
- creating and sticking to an exercise program
- keeping a medication routine
- self-testing your blood sugars
- keeping educated
- getting enough rest
- dealing with the financial implications

Your management plan should be developed with the assistance of members of your management team: family and friends, a physician, a diabetes educator, a pharmacist, a podiatrist, and a dietician who is knowledgeable about diabetes.

That said, the only one who can take the ultimate responsibility is the diabetic himself. There are a few exceptions, of course — children, disabled or very elderly people — but for most people the responsibility lies with themselves. There will be support from family and friends, of course, but ultimately, as they saying goes, the buck stops here.

You, the diabetic, have to take care of you, the person. Look upon it as your maintenance plan. Think about your car, your home. You put gas in your car to make it go. You change the oil filters, rotate the tires, visit your mechanic at signs of problems. You do everything you can to ensure it doesn't break down. Homes get that same level of care, maintenance, and upkeep. You mow the grass, paint the trim, vacuum the floors.

So why on earth would you not do the same thing for yourself? Your body, your own physical and mental well-being, certainly deserves the same amount of time and energy as your car or your home.

Look at your body as a car. You don't want it to break down and leave you with problems to deal with. To keep it in good order, you need to keep your blood sugars close to normal twenty-four hours a day. You need to keep that glucose down because when you have too much it can:

- damage your kidneys and cause kidney disease;
- weaken the blood vessels in the retina of your eye, possibly leading to blindness;
- damage nerves, causing numbness and tingling in hands and feet, problems with digestion, urination, and sexual function, and lead to amputations of the feet;
- speed up normal hardening of the arteries, leading to heart disease and stroke at an earlier age; and
- increase the likelihood for men of developing pancreatic and liver cancer.

The scenario is not all doom and gloom. By being proactive you can gain better control.

- Set goals for effectively managing your diabetes with your physician and diabetes educators and strive every day to meet those goals.
- Know your target numbers and have your blood sugar, cholesterol, blood pressure, and A1C (a calculated average

of your blood glucose levels over the past sixty to ninety days) tested according to the schedule set by your physician.

- Eat well, following the meal plan worked out with your educators. You will learn to appreciate proper foods as a tool to feeling good.
- Keep fit by setting and maintaining your target weight and exercising regularly.
- Take a walk every day, even if it's indoors at the mall or on a track.
- Take all medications exactly as prescribed by your physician.
- Explore the benefits of vitamin supplements and take those appropriate after checking with your doctor.
- Learn to relax. We all know stress can raise blood sugars and just generally create a negative attitude, so learn ways to relax even if you need to seek help to do it.
- Schedule and keep regular eye exams and do everything recommended for your eyes.
- Take care of your feet by learning and practising proper daily foot care routines and by having your feet checked regularly by your doctor or foot care specialist.
- Request regular kidney function tests and checks for kidney disease.
- Be alert for numbness or pins and needles in your hands or feet. Tell your doctor if you experience them.
- Get your meter checked for accuracy at least once a year, or more often if you start to doubt its accuracy.
- Chart when you should have various checks and tests and call your doctor's office to arrange them. These should include HbA1C blood tests and blood pressure measurements every two to four months, kidney checks and foot exams every six to twelve months, annual eye examinations by an eye specialist, and annual or more frequent blood fat tests.
- Take steps to improve your medical care if you are not satisfied with the care you receive. It is your right, so fight for it. We address this in chapter eight.

All of these things work towards maintaining your health, give you the assurance of being in control, take away fears, and prevent many complications that diabetics face.

No matter how many challenges you have, how many difficult times, reading the stories of others always does two things: it makes you aware of positive things in your own situation, and it gives you inspiration to keep plugging, to work for your own health.

A SMALL PRICE TO PAY

AE from British Columbia is a Type 1 diabetic who shared her story because she feels doing so through this book will help a lot of people.

"I was diagnosed when I was fifty-one and instantly insulin dependent. (I am now seventy-five.) I had been on holiday to L.A. and had difficulty reading the big green road signs. When I got home I developed a bellyache. My doctor did a complete blood review and my blood sugar was extremely high. He told me to get to the hospital immediately and they put me on forty-five units of insulin right away.

"Over the next ten years they tried all kinds of different insulin on me but I remained a brittle diabetic; never was able to get good control.

"I developed diabetic neuropathy, extreme pain in both legs, for a year, having to resort to Tylenol 3, which caused constipation. Then a blood vessel broke in my eye and I was sent to a retinologist for many laser treatments over the next ten years.

"Finally Humalog came along and my endocrinologist made up a plan for me: if my blood glucose was between five and seven, I took five Humalog with breakfast. And so on, a plan for lunch and dinner. At nighttime, I still had to take some NPH insulin.

"Often at 2:00 or 3:00 a.m. I would get a hypoglycemic reaction. A few times my husband couldn't wake me and had to call 911. And off to emergency they would take me and give me glucose. Finally, in 2001, the U.S.A. came up with a new insulin, made in Germany, called Lantus. My endocrinologist made arrangements with a pharmacy in Blaine, Washington, to give me two vials of Lantus every four months.

"I take twenty-five units of Lantus at bedtime and there are no more hypoglycemic experiences. I hope someday that Canada will finally be able to supply it to all diabetics. If I had been able to control my diabetes sooner, my vision wouldn't be impaired. However, I can still read large-print books and can still drive to the village, to play bridge, but can't drive on the highway."

When asked what advice she would give to other diabetics, AE said: "I would tell all diabetics to enjoy their fruits and vegetables and forget about desserts. A small price to pay for good health. My husband says he's glad he's on a diabetic diet because he doesn't gain weight! Carry a small bottle of juice and a couple of crackers with you when you go out. Don't leave home without them!"

There is one other thing that she does that others can benefit from: AE enjoys communicating via her computer. To make emailing possible she has turned the size of the type up to larger, bolder print so that she can read it.

OUTLOOK AFFECTS CONTROL; CONTROL AFFECTS OUTLOOK

One thing that was very obvious to me as I interviewed people for this book was that those who have a management plan, who feel in control, are not only handling their disease and in better health, but they also have a much better mental outlook. They are happier people. They have better relationships with family and friends. They are enjoying life more.

The best control is maintained by being organized and following a schedule. A schedule isn't the worst thing in life.

It is usually when their normal routine is changed for some reason that diabetics experience problems. Jack, for instance, has had trouble keeping his routine all summer. We had non-stop company, which makes timing more difficult. He also injured his back, so he was not able to get his usual game of golf or morning skate at the local arena in. In fact, for several weeks he could hardly walk.

"Just being off-schedule like that, I keep bottoming out," he says. "It affects me most in the chest. I get a lot of pain and discomfort."

HYPO OR HYPER?

You might hear the words *hypoglycemia* and *hyperglycemia* from those in the medical profession. The terms can be confusing. Just remember that *hypo* means *less than*. In other words, your blood sugars are less than the safe point. *Hyperglycemia* means that your blood sugars are higher than your target range.

Staying within your target range is very important to your long-term health. It reduces the risk of eye damage, kidney disease, high blood pressure, heart disease and stroke, infections, impotence, and problems with pregnancy.

We all get sick from time to time, for a variety of reasons ranging from bugs to serious illness. Diabetics must take care of their over-all health and test their blood glucose levels more often when they are sick and test for ketones several times a day.

> HYPERGLYCEMIA = high blood glucose or sugar
> HYPOGLYCEMIA = low blood glucose or sugar

LOW BLOOD SUGAR REACTIONS

When blood sugars drop too low a number of symptoms occur, including sweating, trembling, hunger, dizziness, moodiness, confusion, and numbness in the arms or hands.

You will get to know your symptoms. When you experience the symptoms above, step one should be to test your blood to make sure you are indeed experiencing low blood sugar (a.k.a. hypoglycemia, insulin reaction, or insulin shock).

If you are low, immediate steps need to be taken. You should have learned those steps from your diabetes educator. They might include drinking a glass of fast-acting carbohydrate such as a sports drink, orange juice, or a non-diet soft drink; taking fast-dissolving glucose tablets (check the suggested number on the package); or eating some high-sugar food. A small tube of ready-to-use icing, such as Cake Mate, is handy to carry and works well, or try a tablespoon of honey, hard candies, or chocolate. Whatever you use, symptoms should begin to stop after ten to fifteen minutes.

If they don't, further action is needed — more intake of sugar and if necessary a run to the hospital. Ask in your training sessions what to do in this event. Left untreated, hypoglycemia can cause convulsions or unconsciousness. This is why you should always carry your tester and something to treat a low blood sugar reaction. You also must wear Medic-Alert information.

If you have a low blood sugar reaction and your next meal is more than an hour away, then you should eat a snack of some kind, like half a sandwich or cheese and crackers. Something that will "tide you over."

Low blood sugars can be caused by a number of things:

SETTING YOUR TARGETS

Your target range for blood sugar readings should be discussed with your doctor. For most people anything below 4.0 is considered low, and anything above 11.0 is considered high. However, everyone is different, so take note of how you feel at various readings and discuss this with your physician.

If you have Type 2 diabetes and are having trouble reaching or maintaining your targeted blood sugar range you need to take action to correct that. First make an appointment with your doctor, then for a minimum of three days prior to the appointment test your blood sugars regularly — before meals and two hours after your biggest meal. It is also a good idea to test as soon as you get up in the morning. Record these readings in your logbook and take them in to discuss with your doctor.

This is the control you need to maintain to stay feeling your best. By working with a member of your care team you are becoming a management pro.

- taking too much medication
- eating too little food
- not eating on time
- being more physically active than usual
- getting a lot of exercise
- drinking alcohol

It is important to keep track of these lows so that you find your range. Jack has been known to go below 3.0 before he begins to experience the signals. Because of that he is more aware of doing frequent testing. For example he always tests before he drives. He also acts very quickly if he is experiencing symptoms. We both do; if I sense the irritability that is his telltale sign I ask him to check. If he refuses, I insist — that is a sure sign that he is low.

> Speaking of a fellow motorcyclist no longer able to enjoy the lifestyle he loved so much, a rider said, "My buddy was diabetic. He lost both legs. One toe, another toe, a foot, both legs … a piece at a time."
>
> Emotional, he turned away. This biker, who is also diabetic, says seeing what his friend has gone through inspires him to manage his own diabetes and stay on plan.

If you are having lows with any frequency make an appointment to discuss it with your physician.

HIGH BLOOD SUGAR REACTIONS

The signs of high blood sugars are a little different. You may be thirsty, very tired, or urinate more often.

If you are having consistent highs make an appointment to see your doctor. Your medication or insulin may need to be adjusted. You may have to adjust your meals or increase your physical activity.

ONE STORY, TWO PERSPECTIVES

WF of Astorville, Ontario, is a Type 1 diabetic, diagnosed in 1999 when he was fifteen. He takes insulin injections. His diagnosis came about because he was "constantly feeling very sick and dehydrated, being unable to eat. Very moody, constantly thirsty."

Reading the story from WF's perspective you get the impression that he has his diabetes well in hand and is controlling his life well. But he's a teenager. His mother's perspective is very different and gives a picture of stress felt by a parent. After all, they have to add concerns about his long-term health to the normal angst of parenting a teen.

The Younger Perspective

WF says the biggest challenge he faces is keeping on top of his diabetes while trying to lead a normal life. "You almost need to choose between a diabetic life and a normal one. It's difficult to combine the two. It is lots of work to take care of yourself and maintain good numbers.

"The hardest is keeping up good habits. Unless you have a very repetitive schedule, it's hard to balance insulin with carbohydrates while keeping your blood sugar in mind. When you are really hungry, you don't want to spend your time counting carbohydrates and figuring out how much insulin the meal requires.

"I know that diabetic supplies are very expensive, and I feel guilty because my parents are paying for them. I'm nineteen years old, and there is no way I could afford them right now. I know it isn't my fault that I am diabetic, but you can't help feel like a burden when you are costing your family so much."

WF has a few tips to pass along. "A backpack is good for carrying diabetic supplies and candy in case of a low blood sugar. A mini cooler is good method to carry extra cartridges of insulin if you're travelling long distances."

He says anyone newly diagnosed with diabetes must give it time. "It feels very foreign at first, but after about the first year of being a diabetic it seems very normal. You almost forget what it was like living before diabetes. There are much worse diseases to live with. I remember lying in a hospital bed after first being diagnosed surrounded by very sick children and feeling as though I didn't belong there. Diabetes can be very irritating, but at least you can still maintain a fairly normal lifestyle compared to many other sicknesses."

We asked if there was anything he would like to say to those close to him who are affected by the disease. "My parents are constantly worried about my health. I feel I could be taking better care of myself for them, because they are very supportive. I think it actually affects them more than it does me. I think they would worry regardless of my habits, though, because they are not living with diabetes first-hand. There is no way to explain the feeling of a very bad low blood sugar without experiencing it. It's hard to understand something you haven't experienced. My mother suffers from a sickness as well, and I'm not going to pretend I know what it's like, because I don't. I worry about her, but without fully understanding it. I think diabetes is the same."

A Parent's Perspective

This young man's mother, K.F. gave us her perspective on her son's disease. "My son is a Type 1 diabetic who was diagnosed around his fifteenth birthday. He takes four injections of insulin a day. At the time he was diagnosed, I was very concerned that he was dying. He was very ill and very thin. He had gone from active to inactive and his rib cage had become very deformed. When the classic symptoms of diabetes (consuming massive quantities of liquid and frequent urination) arose, I recognized them and got him to the nearest walk-in clinic. (We were living in Alberta at the time.)

"Unfortunately, the whole west end of the city had a blackout while we sat in the waiting room. We were ushered into the doctor's office, regardless of the lack of light. When I expressed my theory, the doctor exclaimed my son could not possibly have diabetes because he didn't look sick enough. He was peering at my son with a pen flashlight, and they were unable to give him a blood test due to the blackout. I insisted that he did have diabetes, so he reluctantly said, 'Bring him back in the morning, and we'll run a blood test.' By one o'clock the next day my son and I were both sitting in the hospital (alongside a sheepish doctor) waiting for my son's first insulin injection. This was followed up by a long week of diabetic training for the whole family.

"There are good things about being diagnosed with Type 1 diabetes at fifteen. My son had enjoyed the childhood freedom of spontaneous eating and living in those carefree years. He had had his share of gathering treats he could eat freely at Halloween, Christmas, and Easter. At fifteen, he did not even flinch at getting his injections or testing his blood like many younger children do. Most of the diabetic responsibility got handed over to him right away.

"On the down side, these were his growth years; his body was already fighting a hormonal battle. Even with the proper amounts of insulin, he felt poorly much of the time. He had something called sliding rib syndrome wherein one side of your rib cage grows at a different rate than the other side.

"Frequently, he would get sharp pains in his rib cage that would bring him to his knees. It took a long time to figure out what was going on concerning these pains. Much of the food he ate made him feel ill. Soon they were testing him for celiac disease. The idea of having further restrictions on his eating made my son very depressed. However, after much testing, the outcome was that hormonal factors blended with getting the right insulin doses were responsible for these feelings of ill health. When he stopped growing, he felt better. Being a newly diagnosed diabetic did complicate these growing years.

"My son is nineteen now. This is indeed the scary part. He's gone from a model diabetic to someone who wants to have a life despite his diabetes. When he wasn't feeling well, he had monotonous diet and a low-key life. His pediatrician used to tease him about having good numbers in his logbook because he didn't do anything or go anywhere. His three-month A1C was in the good range most of the time. Later that year, we finally sold our house, and we moved to northern Ontario.

"Here, he met other diabetic teens who stopped going to the diabetes centres because 'they didn't like the flack' when their numbers were not good. Some of the more rebellious ones talked about highs and lows like other teens talk about getting wasted at a Saturday night party. Soon the 'teen brain,' which can't get all excited about what could happen to them down the road, kicked in. I assume that many of the diabetic teens live like many non-diabetic teens are living (like we all did) for the here and now. They feel not only invincible but unconcerned about the future. If bad numbers made your face turn purple instantly or your ears fall off, there might be more of a concern about bad numbers, but the complications are years off.

"My son moved away from home right after high school to have a life. He no longer weighs food or reads the labels to find out about the carb count. He takes his insulin after meals if he remembers. He stopped going to the diabetes centre. The doctor he sees now does not seem to get too excited if his A1C is in the high range. Occasionally, a very high reading will get my son back on track for several days, but then he gets much too casual again. My biggest fear is that he likes to drink alcohol, and that he may take his nighttime insulin twice on a night that he has had a little too much rum. Though every person who lives with or cares about a diabetic gets concerned about a high blood sugar reading, we all know that too much insulin can result in a coma and/or sudden death.

"The biggest frustration is talking to someone who refuses to listen or trying to get to sleep when they've been out to a party and forgot to call you to let you know where they are even bedding down for the night. These are regular problems with many teenagers, but worse when your teen is diabetic. You not only worry about the drinking and drugs but the food and the insulin. You find yourself getting uptight at a family meal when he starts eating without testing his blood and then shoots up some random number of insulin based on what?

"You wonder, if they are this slack around you, what is it like back at their place with all their non-diabetic friends around? Or worse still, when there is nobody around. My son is no dummy. He finished high school with honours and is presently attending a good college with hopes of a bright future ahead of him. He is a social being with numerous talents. He doesn't seem to worry about being accepted, he just gets accepted by most people who know him. So where is this coming from? Of course, being his mother, I feel responsible for his health, but since he left home, it is out of my hands. I keep wondering, if he had've got diabetes when he was younger, and I had've had a few more years with him at home, would that have made a difference to his diabetic habits?

"I feel like my son and I have a great relationship when we avoid the diabetes issue. However, I know being able to chat and joke with someone while avoiding this issue is not really much of a relationship. It's a relationship based on looking the other way. I hate to say that sometimes I feel that this is the only relationship we can have at this point. When I can lighten up about the situation, I tell him, 'I plan on not getting too attached to you!'

"My advice is that very weary, overdone chestnut: be there for them. Lately, I am seeing signs that he's thinking a little more about his promising future and this includes his health issues. The rebel side of his being is giving way to someone who wants to make a mark. I'm not holding my breath, but I'm trying not to wreck my life by worrying excessively about him. (Ha! Not easily done!) He has an older brother and a father who care deeply about him. We all have to hope that his 'having a life' doesn't mean losing it too soon to diabetic complications."

This mother's story is one that wrenched at my heart, for she is such a true example of the impact this disease has on those who love a diabetic. The level of impact is one that no diabetic should ignore. If they care at all about those around them, then they need to consider the impact their actions have on others.

CHAPTER 3
Impact on Others

Interesting experience today. Here we are in a favourite restaurant. Jack is face down on the table. Sitting across from a man with his head down on the table is a little disconcerting. Waitresses and other patrons are concerned, of course. So am I. Certainly it isn't an enjoyable experience for any of us. I'm sure they all wonder at me, calmly writing in my notebook.

Today is a real example of him pushing himself too hard and getting into trouble. He got out of the hospital last night and insisted that he wanted to go out for breakfast today. After living on the hospital version of a diabetic diet for eleven days he wanted real food. I offered to cook him breakfast at home, but no, he wanted to go out. So out we went.

Our perfectly poached eggs haven't arrived yet, but I'm pretty sure it's not low sugars that have him kissing the table. He tested 5.5 before we left home just twenty minutes before. He is just too darn weak to be gallivanting about after the rough stint he had in the hospital. Weak he may be, but he is still stubborn. It takes me back to the days before the pump, actually before insulin, when eating on time was so vitally important.

In one memorable incident, we had been invited to a reception where a hockey star was to be the featured guest. Jack's mother was visiting and was a real fan, so we decided to go. As a journalist I get invited to many occasions like this, but normally Jack doesn't go with me — the timing and the food just don't work for him, and he doesn't particularly enjoy schmoozing. This event, to be held at the poshest hotel in town, was not only luring us with the hockey guy, but it was also billed as a showcase of local seafood. Very appealing.

So, at about five o'clock I started to get supper for Jack. His normal eating time was five-thirty and he had to eat by six or he'd be in trouble. But the boy didn't want to admit to that this day because his mother was visiting. No, we would eat at the reception. It was due to start at seven o'clock. My gut told me trouble was brewing, but I let myself be manipulated. I didn't want to create a fuss.

We arrived early. Not easy because Mom always likes to take her time, have another beer, and make an entrance after things have warmed up. I had been pushing because I knew Jack needed to get food into him. I had been trying for some time to get him to eat a sandwich or an apple. By seven o'clock he was starting to exhibit the unreasonable, irritable behaviour that is so typical of a diabetic out of whack.

He was determined to wait. Finally the food arrived. It was now seven-thirty or later. The food was exactly what you'd expect at a classy reception in a fine-dining establishment. Excellent nibbles. But for a diabetic it was all "over prepared" in rich sauces — oysters smothered with cheese, that sort of thing. His nibs ate a few steamed mussels, but generally was, by now, so irritable that he simply refused all of the other things he could have had. Veggies, cheese, crackers, and fruits were all on trays. And there was a variety of seafood as well as rolls. It was no longer about the food. It was about Jack with low sugars being as stubborn as hell.

The evening was becoming a nightmare for me. Do I nag and risk a scene in a place where I need to make a good impression for the sake of my career? Or do I ignore him, knowing he's getting himself into trouble? I opted for getting out and away from there, although I knew I should stay to meet people important to my work. As much as I knew he needed to eat, I also knew that his irritability could result in an outburst that could have worse implications.

Since Mother had her autographed picture of the hockey guy, and I had taken their photo, and she had consumed a couple of beers, and she didn't like seafood anyway, I devised a plan. She was annoyed. She was having a good time and the beer was free. Jack was not going to do anything I suggested. That's when my militant side kicked in.

"Come on, let's go to Harvey's. I want some real food." Jack loves this hamburger joint's fare and I figured he would eat there. I gave Mother the option of coming with us or taking a taxi home. She came with us.

"I'm driving," I announced, and I didn't waste any time. By the time we went into the fast food joint Jack was pretty shaky. I sat him and his mother at a table near the door and rushed up to the counter. Picture the scenario. I'm usually pretty mild tempered and tend to keep the peace rather than make waves — but I've learned to take control when I have to.

"I need orange juice," I said.

"Oh, we only serve juice for breakfast," said the kid behind the counter.

Just then I heard Jack's mother, calling me. "Julie, Julie, there is something wrong with Jack."

Duh!

Teeth gritted, I looked at the kid and spat out, "Get me orange juice now!"

He went over to the pop dispenser and started to pour an orange pop.

"Dammit, get me orange juice or call an ambulance."

Eyes popping out of his head, he went out back and got an orange juice. "That's ninety-nine cents," he said.

I grabbed the juice, threw him five dollars, and said, "I'll be back."

By the time I got to Jack he was face down on the table and pretty unresponsive. I lifted his head, stuck the straw in his mouth, and started my all-too-familiar routine of trying to bring him around.

Shake his shoulders. "Jack, drink some juice."

Shake harder. "Jack, suck on the straw."

Pat his face. "Jack, you have to drink."

All the time my voice was getting louder. He took a couple of pulls on the straw but not enough.

Propping him up in the seat, I shook him hard and my face pats got stronger.

"Jack, drink! Suck the straw."

"Don wanna," he slurred.

"You drink or I'm calling the ambulance." Now I was yelling. A small crowd was gathering. That threat worked. I managed to get the whole container of juice into him by repeating the threat of the ambulance until it was gone. Then I let his head back down onto the table and went and ordered our food. I stared the kid in the face as I placed the order.

"This is what I want. And I want it fast."

"Yes, ma'am," he gulped.

I headed back to the table to calm my now crying mother-in-law and try to bring Jack back to us. When the counter kid called our number I just turned around, gave him the glare, and he delivered our food. It took a half-hour for Jack to come around and eat a bit of food. Longer before he was with it enough to make his way to the car.

Not long after this incident the decision was made that Jack needed to go on insulin.

This situation is an exaggerated example of what can happen when a diabetic gets too low. It is completely true, but thankfully it doesn't happen often. It isn't fun for anyone concerned. For me it is very difficult. It turns me into a nagging bitch. It took my pleasure out of what could have been a very enjoyable evening. It made Jack ill — the effects of this kind of incident don't disappear instantly and have long-reaching implications.

It scared my mother-in-law. It probably had a negative impact on my freelance writing career. It scared me. I hate being set up to be the heavy. Frankly, the one difference between me and many other caregivers of diabetics is that I am too darn loyal and love the guy too much to walk. Many do.

When we married I was not a dominating, militant woman. I was indecisive, shy, and introverted. I was scared a lot of the time. Scared of not being liked, of making a fool of myself, that people would look at me.

Things have changed a lot. My mother often comments to me now that she doesn't understand how I've managed to become so take-charge, to make it as a writer, to care so much about people. It's because I've had to. Like so many others who are coping with having a diabetic to care for I've had to learn to be strong.

Diabetes, without a doubt, has changed my life. Many of my aspirations and dreams have been shelved. Sometimes it's been a hard decision for me. Do I pursue the career I wanted and had started to develop? Do I sacrifice Jack's health and well-being to chase an uncertain life as a food and travel writer? Do I strain my marriage? Can I handle the stress of trying to have everything I want, while still being the wife, mother, and daughter than I strive to be? How can I ensure that our son is not affected by this, that it doesn't affect his relationship with his father? That, for me, was a major concern.

Don't get me wrong — all is not bad. In fact, I think we are far luckier than many. This fight has made us stronger. It's given us the ability to appreciate things that others don't even see. I think I really needed to point out the challenges facing those around the diabetic so that others, too, can find strength together. Looking back on many of the incidents we've faced and overcome we can have a good laugh, share a smile and a wry shake of our heads. Jack's diabetes has brought us closer together. We are a team, best friends, and very comfortable together.

Living with diabetes has given us a different perspective on life. We both value things we didn't even see before. We don't put off things that we want to see or do if we can avoid it. We can't do everything we want; finances won't allow that. But we try to give our lives value. We treasure our families and friends. We consciously try to live a healthier life.

I'm so glad that today's improved treatment of diabetes means increasingly fewer incidents like those at the beginning of this chapter. But they can still happen. People with diabetes really need to acknowledge the effects that they, their disease, and their actions have on other people.

IRRITABLE — NOT ME!

I remember reading a headline on a "Dear Abby" column some years ago. It read "Diabetics Claim Blood Sugar Levels Affect Personality," and a number of letters backed up the statement. Apparently an expert from the American Diabetes Association had tried to say that the disease did not cause irrational, irresponsible, and even violent behaviour. Abby had a flood of letters from people vouching that blood sugar levels can and do affect a person's personality. Many of them were from diabetics who acknowledged what happened to them and their inability at the time to stop it.

Any spouse of a diabetic will confirm that there are times when that is indeed what happens. Never, in our case, the violent behaviour. We had a few moments of irresponsible behaviour in the early days, but no longer. The one thing I thank heaven for every day is that my spouse has accepted responsibility for his disease, recognizes the signs of low and high blood sugars, and acts to do something about it.

It took time. In the early days when he was out of control he would refuse juice or sugar when he went low. He got stubborn and, yes, irrational. I remember once he was going low and decided to go to bed instead of having juice. He had come in late from shoeing horses, hadn't eaten, and was very tired. I saw him staggering and slurring his words; he was annoying and irritable. He started up the stairs in our old farmhouse, with me behind him pushing him forward so that he would fall onto the stairs and not backwards and down them. He crawled up the last few steps and flopped onto the floor of the landing.

I got juice and started the battle to get him to drink it. That was the first time I slapped his face to get him to drink. Not hard, but not a love pat, either. He was out of it for almost half an hour. We lived a good half-hour drive from the hospital, and I was panicking about how I could get him to the car when he finally came around.

We had a discussion after that, and he promised that if I said he was irritable, or if he felt irritable or out of sorts, he would test. Thankfully he has kept that promise.

One of the letters in that "Dear Abby" column said the spouses, partners, and relatives of diabetics are unsung heroes, and that regardless of the greatest challenges faced by diabetics, those who love them are also confronted by trials.

That column held special meaning for me. It confirmed my own conclusions. I kept it to share with others. It is really important for both diabetics and those around them to acknowledge that blood sugars can affect mood, make a person irritable, and even make tempers flare. If you understand what is going on, that it is a diabetic reaction rather than actual anger or meanness directed at you, it makes it easier to deal with.

HOME WORK AND CARE MAKE FOR IFFY BUSINESS

If ever there is a person dealing with more than her fair share of challenges and just plain hard knocks it is CK of Nova Scotia. When I met CK it was like meeting a kindred spirit. I just wanted to fall into her arms and give her a hug. So many things she said hit home.

Like myself, she chose self-employment as a way to be near to her spouse and earn money as well. Also like me, she has a real problem making people understand and respect that she works and is responsible for providing much-needed income as well as support and care. That said, I have to tell you that CK is dealing with a far more difficult situation than I am and she is doing it without a lot of support.

"There are support groups out there, but who can find the time to travel to meetings?" she said.

We both met the love of our lives at a young age and married early. But when she walked down the aisle she had no idea of the hand that life would deal her.

We met at a craft fair where she was selling distressed primitive folk art and pine furniture. She described her wares as "recycled church bits in funky folk art." "See that tin? It's from an old church ceiling. We do mostly pine furniture from January to May, then in May people go back outdoors, so we switch to funky folk art." With a grin she gestures to the handcrafted items, saying, "We put the fun into funky."

During a lull in customers she settled back to share her life experiences. Her story began more than thirty years ago when the couple exchanged marriage vows at the age of eighteen. Six months later, BK, a logger, broke his back while working in the woods. He's been a paraplegic ever since.

In spite of his injuries, complications that have plagued them, and the onset of his diabetes, the couple raised three children. BK began working with wood and CK went into the craft business. Their three children are now grown and away from home.

Rather than life getting easier without children to raise, CK, the caregiver, finds it harder now. In fact sometimes she wonders how she will carry on.

Her story: BK was on two different insulins trying to stay in control, but his injuries, medications, and complications made it very difficult. "He just decided not to take medicine and now controls it with diet. He overdoses with vegetables and fruits. We decided to work one or the other. Cut out red meat. Have a lot of fresh vegetables.

"[My husband] stays with blood sugar around 11.0. That's normal for him. He's very active with his upper-body strength. That helps him stay in control. He's up and down in his chair many times a day. It's like a normal person walking ten miles a day.

"Several other family members have diabetes. His dad is also diabetic. He controls with diet and pills. He's seventy-six. He has prostate cancer. He says he is so conflicted: 'If I eat a diabetic diet then I'm worrying about cancer. If eat the diet for cancer, then I worry about diabetes. It's a vicious circle.' It's a hard go."

Although there is a family history of diabetes, CK believes that her husband wouldn't be diabetic if he were not paralyzed and speculates that the trauma he experienced triggered the disease.

Some of the reality of her life surfaces when another craftswoman who also travels the circuit came over to inform me that "she's an angel."

CK looked me in the eye and with a wry smile said there are times when she would like to chuck it all in. Like many diabetics, BK is subject to moods that are becoming increasingly hard for CK to deal with.

"I'm a positive, optimistic person. He started as a craftsperson. Helped to raise our three kids. We raised them on less than seven thousand dollars a year. We spent time together, travelled, enjoyed life. But there are times when his moods are bad.... He had a hard time growing up and it seems to be coming back to him now.

"We've gone through a lot. It's been awful at times, but you pick yourself up and go on. I can hear my mother, on a daily basis: 'You get off your butt if you want this to work.' I have to be positive, upbeat, and optimistic all the time. I'm like that.

"BK is pessimistic, negative. He's opposite. That causes some tense and frustrating moments. We've been married thirty years. Now he's started getting verbally abusive."

While she knows and understands that many factors are responsible, including the stress his body is under and his diabetes, she says she began having panic attacks when she was thirty and has trouble sleeping.

"It gets overwhelming."

She says one of their biggest challenges is financial. BK gets compensation and disability pay, but it's been taking all of his money to buy supplies.

"This is my business," she says, gesturing to the crafts and furniture in her booth. Although the craft business has been excellent for the couple in terms of flexible hours, allowing them to work at home and together at something, the uncertainty of cash flow makes it difficult. "It's an iffy business, like gambling."

When they travel to craft shows they camp in their van or in a tent until the snow flies, and then they use hotels. Costs are increasing dramatically both for the business and in their daily lives. To help her sleep, CK turns to inexpensive medications such as cheap travel sickness pills.

Another challenge for her is making people take her dedication to her business and her need to work to maintain their income seriously. Their two dads are alone. "We watch for them, build stuff at

BK's dad's so we can watch over him. He just thinks I'm his cook and housekeeper. My dad thinks I don't work. He wants me to travel."

CK finds that having her own business allows her to be close to her diabetic husband and father-in-law. She also highly values the joy she gets from what she does.

"Craft work is relaxing — I love to paint and create stuff." Her funky folk art is, for her, fun both in the creating and in the selling.

Most importantly, she says, "If you love each other enough, believe in each other enough, it all works out."

CK is a woman whose life has been fully impacted by more than one medical challenge. The way she and her husband worked together to build a life is an inspiration. I can relate to his negative personality. Jack tends to be the same at times, while I'm a disgustingly cheerful optimist.

I also admire the fact that they found a business that allows her to be there for him, for them to work together, to have goals together. Although his extreme medical situation is causing more and more problems now, and CK is frustrated by her current situation, the early days of his diagnosis were handled well as a couple.

JM of Prince Edward Island is another woman who found herself angry and upset with how her husband handled his diagnosis. Her situation has now improved, but she admits to feeling dismayed that her husband is no longer the man she married.

TOUGH LOVE APPROACH PAYS OFF

The moment JM started talking it was obvious that she was angry and upset with her husband. He had refused to look after himself when he was first diagnosed, and that hurt her. She was at the end of her tether with him and the stress he put on the rest of the family. I had told her how I think diabetes is a family disease and that many diabetics, especially men, who would never do anything to harm their family, suddenly do. They put stress on everyone and upset the household. People worry. She jumped right in and was quite emotional.

"My husband never took ownership of his diabetes when diagnosed. I did everything for him. It really took a toll on me. My uncle was dying of the same thing — end stage diabetes. When he [her husband] was diagnosed with heart disease in July he wouldn't do anything to make it better. He kept doing all the things that had made him sick. In January he was facing open-heart surgery. I said to him I couldn't keep on that way. He had a lot of anger because he is sick and I'm healthy."

It took some tough love and a few reality checks, but her husband, with the help of his wife and physician, has changed his attitude and is taking responsibility for his own health and how his actions affect those around him.

"I put it to him, he had to change. I told him it was a slow form of suicide," she says. "Now he's taking charge, testing every morning. His heart doctor was really good. He said to him, if you want to work with me I'll work with you. But if not, there are a lot of people who need me and who are willing to look after themselves."

The doctor forced him to make the decision — to work with him or leave. Fortunately he chose to develop a management plan, to get in control.

"He's really improved," she says. "He doesn't drink like he used to, is watching what he eats. He accepted ownership. He realized, if I take care of myself it will be better. It's easier for me now.

"As women we are used to taking care of ourselves and our families. He had to learn to take care of himself. It's harder for a man to be sick."

The kind of support that JM received from her husband's doctor is a great example of how a team can work together. It's easy to buck against one person, but when a number of people are reinforcing the others' messages, they do have a better chance of sinking in.

When talking to diabetic families they almost universally have nothing but praise for their doctors, educators, nurses, and specialists. They also, almost universally, express a great deal of frustration about the lack of communication between these individuals on their management team. We all know that medical professionals can't hold our hands all the time, but consulting with each other about treatments, how things interact, or how a treatment by one specialist affects something being done by another are vital components of proper health care that many of us fear might fall through the cracks.

Spouses often find themselves in a position of having to carry information from one specialist to another. Or of having to say, "But so and so said this or that." It can be scary. One diabetic complained recently of a specialist for a bowel disorder — whom he had waited months to see — prescribing a drug that made him ill. He read the label, and it said very clearly, "Not to be taken if you have diabetes." Because he did not have a regular pharmacist, the error was not caught. He not only suffered the side effects for a few rough days, he now has to try to get a different medication, further delaying treatment.

People also have to face learning on the job, so to speak. To seek out the correct information as it applies to their particular case, to be knowledgeable enough to be protective, to know what signals trouble, what to do, and how to cope often falls to the family.

As one mother said, "[Diabetes] is an epidemic," and yet knowledge in the community of the needs of diabetics and their families is lacking, and because of that, so is the support that is sometimes craved.

FACING THE FEARS — ONE DAY AT A TIME

DOH's twelve-year-old daughter is an insulin-dependent Type 1 diabetic.

"As a mother, I can't help but worry and be scared. As my daughter gets older and starts to care for herself, I am reminded that low blood sugars can impair the judgment of an individual. It's one thing to let your child ride her bike to school, but it's another knowing that children could wander off disorientated if they don't treat their low blood sugar conditions.

"There's also a great deal of confusion between the care for someone with Type 1 diabetes and Type 2. It's much easier [with Type 1] to miscalculate the insulin dosage or even make errors by accidentally switching and administering the wrong insulin. I'll never forget the time we made that error and had to force our daughter to eat three full meals in the space of an hour. We could have lost her, but once you face death head on and survive, you do learn to relax, as you build strength from your experiences.

"Also, caring for a child with diabetes has different concerns and stresses than living with a husband or sibling who is old enough to care for themselves. However, I imagine once long-term complications set in, then the fear returns. We already know of one family whose son lost the use of his eyes, and just recently another family buried their thirty-plus-year-old due to severe complications associated with living with diabetes. You live with the philosophy 'one day at a time.' Make the most of every moment because you don't know what is around the corner."

She says that there have been many frustrating aspects of having a diabetic in her life. "Initially, trying to give a needle to a crying child was frustrating and heartbreaking at the same time. Not having family close by was another problem because the extra hands would have lessened the stress by allowing my husband and me to have a break. Counting carbohydrates and measuring food, living in the kitchen and handing out snacks was never a picnic for me. Now we're over that.

"Today the frustration comes from those who belittle the condition and aren't willing to walk in our shoes and listen to our concerns. The public thinks they know what diabetes is, but there are major differences between what someone with Type 1 deals with versus someone with Type 2. You just can't lump them in the same category. Also, the concern for diabetes tends to be over-shadowed by other conditions such as cancer, heart disease, and stroke. Many people don't realize that once a person gets diabetes their chances of having circulatory and heart problems increases."

Children are affected by diabetes in more ways than one. We've had several people tell their stories of dealing with childhood diabetes, but what about children who have a diabetic parent?

On July 16, 2004, a news item on CTV's *Canada AM* related the tale of a four-year-old girl who was being hailed as a hero. She had found her mother unconscious — in a diabetic coma — and called 911. She told them her address and said her mommy's sugars were low.

Help arrived and her mom received treatment. She had been unconscious for over an hour.

Here is a typical case of a family where the child was aware and, thanks to her parents, knew what to do. When asked if they taught her about diabetes, her mom said from the time her daughter was about two she had had problems and been sick. They tried to reinforce with the child that 911 was the number to call if she needed help.

Although the little girl was said to be mature for her age, the reality is that she has had to learn to cope, how to handle the fact that her mom is sick and sometimes has problems. Thanks to this little girl, her mom survived.

This speaks of a strong family fortunate to have a wonderful daughter with the necessary knowledge to handle a frightening situation when it arose. To my mind this is also one fortunate little girl. She is going to grow into a strong adult because she is learning how to cope.

NO VACATION FROM DIABETES

BM of New Brunswick has the double worry of having two diabetics in her family. Having coped with her husband's disease she now worries about her son, who is finding his way in life.

"Because my husband doesn't cook and, in the early years of our marriage, had little knowledge of nutrition, I feel responsible for providing proper balanced meals that meet his diabetic needs. I don't 'police' his portions or snacks, just make sure appropriate food is available.

"There can be no vacation from diabetes because mealtimes can't fluctuate much and food must always be available. Very few foods are free, even on vacations.

"No matter how independent a person with diabetes is, he must always be aware of the risk of a severe hypoglycemic reaction which requires assistance. My husband has had many reactions in his sleep which required my assistance — occasionally with glucagon. Therefore I hesitate to be away overnight. And for many years I worked shifts and was away all night.

"Several times he has been close to unconsciousness, and I was frightened that I wouldn't be able to get him back, but always knowing that 911 was an option.

"Much worse than that was my fear for my son as he struggled to lead an independent, active life away from us. Wilderness camping, planting trees in the Rockies, working on a fish farm in the ocean. Knowing he could need help and have no one there to give it.

"The most frustrating aspect of life with a diabetic is that sometimes things don't go as they should [with blood sugars] no matter how hard you try. Plans must be changed; meals aren't eaten. Everything must revolve around mealtimes. Travelling with other people is difficult.

"It is easier for me to run interference for my diabetics than it is for them. Rather than ask others to change their plans when they conflict with the diabetic's needs, he will jeopardize his health to avoid drawing attention to himself.

"When the children were young, often their needs and wants had to take second place to the diabetes. At times I was frustrated and resentful, then felt guilty because it's not my husband's fault that he has diabetes.

"When I consider my son's lot in life, I often feel so upset for him, knowing what he misses out on and how his health will suffer as he ages, but also proud of the way he handles his disease and its restrictions.

"Just now, my husband has developed unstable angina due to coronary artery disease as a direct result of his diabetes. His cholesterol levels and blood pressure are within the set parameters because of medication and his compliance with diet, etc. He has no risk factors *except* forty-eight years of insulin-dependent diabetes. Not his fault!

"It makes me fear for my son. And it is a worry for me and my husband. But we manage by constantly being aware of the constrictions and requirements."

ADULT CHILDREN WITH DIABETIC PARENTS

KV of Ontario worries about her diabetic mother. "My mom was diagnosed with Type 2 diabetes last year, and I went with her to the nutritional counselling sessions. I've been very concerned because she seems to be in denial about her disease, ordering regular pop and dessert with dinner at restaurants, forgetting to take her pills with her on vacation, etc. I've gone so far as to chase after waiters and ask them to give my mom something other than what she ordered. It makes everyone feel like garbage, and I have to say I'm starting to feel resentful that she's not taking her disease seriously. At the same time I can only imagine how hard it is for her."

HIDING THE WORRY

Sometimes adult children with diabetes hide their disease to protect a parent. VM from Ontario writes, "One of our challenges has been to hide the effects of the disease from my husband's aging parents while still trying to impress upon them that he needs to eat on time and to stay away from traditional rich, sweet foods.

"I'm always tense when we visit. I know that he's making himself ill because he doesn't want to upset them. They have lost other children and are feeling very vulnerable because of their own health problems. I feel bad for them and always feel guilty when we leave for home.

"It's hard for me. I know he'll be sick after we leave. Sometimes he can't even drive home. He's all off his program. He hasn't done his shots for fear they would see.

"He seems to accept that he has to manage his food and shots until he goes home to his mom and dad's. There he goes into total denial that he's a diabetic.

"It's really hard. I seem to always be the one who has to cope. I have to cover for him when I phone in because he's too sick to go to work. My stomach is in knots because I'm afraid they will say, every time he takes vacation time, he's sick and can't come back to work on time. We can't pay him.

"I don't know how much longer I can be here. Until the kids finish school, I guess."

VM's letter demonstrates the stress many feel when their diabetic spouse is in denial. They feel like they're burning out, being put upon and under-appreciated. My message to those people is that it is important that you look after yourself, the caregiver, as well as the patient.

Many of us, particularly women, tend to turn up our nurturing instinct and take on responsibility for far too much. In talking to people for this book, I've had dozens of men say to me, "Oh, I let my wife worry about that. She takes care of me." If anything ever happened to the little woman they would, they admit, be in big trouble.

We once sat in an education session with a couple just a few years older than we are. The diabetic man had been brought in to try to get him to change some of his bad habits. As far as he was concerned, cooking and meals and all that stuff were his wife's jobs. He worked in the construction business, working with heavy equipment and such.

In one breath he complained that he couldn't adjust his schedule to worry about things like eating on time. Nor could he give up his sweets or his cigarettes. In the next breath he complained about feeling poorly and said if this was how he was to live his life then he didn't want anything to do with it. He was just going to have his drink, smoke his cigarette, and eat his pie because they were the only things he enjoyed in life, and without them he just didn't want to be here.

His wife sat at the table, eyes down, obviously trying to hold back her tears. I often think about them and wonder if he has any concept of how much he hurt his wife with that statement. He cast her off as nothing. He publicly announced that a piece of pie and a drag on a cigarette meant more to him than she did. Even though she stuck with him for forty-five years, looked after him and took on responsibility for trying to keep him healthy, he didn't for one minute consider the impact his actions had on her.

The instructor and I looked at each other and shook our heads. It was sad. I only hope that she looks after herself and builds a life for herself aside from looking after him. I often think of that woman and wish I could extend a helping hand to her. Unfortunately I didn't get her address, and she is in another province.

The sacrifices of caregivers cannot be measured. But they can be acknowledged.

I do without a lot. It seems that every time I need something, like new glasses, new insoles for my shoes, a new winter coat, boots, or even a simple treat for myself like a good book or a weekend away, there is something Jack needs. He is the first person to tell me to get what I need, to do what I want to do. He's terrific and generous. However, I am always so aware of his health. His eyes are so critical. Mine are okay. A diabetic's feet are a danger zone. My feet are okay; I can make do. Because of his poor circulation he feels the cold so much. I can get another winter out of my jacket. How can I waste money on a book or time away when it could be spent on his health care and comfort?

I'm not by any stretch of the imagination a martyr. I do lots of things for myself and work hard to maintain my lifestyle. I also have a very supportive husband. But at the same time, for me, his health is number one. In our case we have a decent income. We have health insurance that covers our drugs.

One of the things that we have found to work for us is acknowledging each other: "Hey, hon, I'm under the weather. Sorry you have to take on all of the chores." Then a few days later he will take over for me because I have deadlines or things I want to do. He will get the meals, walk the dog, do the dishes, vacuum. "It's my turn," he'll say. "You go ahead and work." The fact that I work at home as a writer/publisher/craftsperson/consultant allows us this flexibility.

There is a tendency in some of us to try to do it all. Natural caregivers, we take on the task of managing the health of our significant others, taking on more and more responsibility. The concern is always that caregivers tend to neglect themselves. The answer is not to stop. We know that those with a nurturing nature simply cannot just give up on someone they love, nor would we expect them to. The aim is to find balance. What we do hope is that you will realize the importance of maintaining your own health and well-being as well as that of those around you.

"ME TIME"

It is really important for all of us to take some "me time." One good way is to start taking fifteen minutes or half an hour for yourself each day. I can hear the arguments already: I don't have time. I don't need it. It won't work. I have to watch the kids.

We're not listening. It is my theory that you need to take a bit of your time as transition time. Let me give you an example. I work at home. I'm a writer and have been able to make a living at this uncertain business because I'm disciplined. My husband is exceptionally good about helping around the house now that he is retired, but there are times when I have to take over.

So I developed a system for those days that basically works for me. I'm an early riser. I take the dog for a tinkle, feed her, feed me, feed Jack if need be, do a bit of housework — all first thing. I try to get the necessary things out of the way before sitting down in my office.

My work requires me to focus. I need to shed the daily worries and things that I know should be done. My method? Once those necessary household things are done I call the dog, grab my book, and head out for a walk in the fields near our house. There is a fallen tree up on a hill, so I aim for that. I usually get only ten minutes to read before the dog is demanding my attention to important matters like throwing an apple from a nearby tree (her favourite chasing thing) or going exploring. Half an hour later I'm refreshed in body from the exercise and my mind has had time to move from household concerns and turn to working things.

Some of my best writing and creativity comes after these walks. I carry a notepad and pen in case inspiration strikes or to make a note of something that needs doing. That seems to allow me to relax and focus even more.

People who work away from home can be seen making their transition by stopping for a coffee. Fifteen minutes with the paper or some conversation is wonderful. When I worked away from home I had a fairly stressful job that was hard to leave behind. I used to pull off the highway into a scenic lookout and just sit for ten minutes.

A friend uses visual imaging — she has a favourite chair where she sits, eyes closed, feet up, and conjures up favourite memories: a visit from her kids, a vacation, a lunch with her sisters. Another friend takes a few minutes, locked in the bathroom, to read a chapter of her book.

The important thing is to recognize that you are taking a few minutes of "me time." Women in particular tend to juggle so many things in their day that they can end up feeling drained. Think of "me time" as your energy builder.

LAUGHTER IS GOOD MEDICINE

Another thing that we all need in our lives is the ability to laugh, a sense of humour. Jack and I often have people comment on our ability to laugh and joke our way through some of the bad times. Even during a crisis — in a hospital emergency room or when dealing with worries of some kind — we are usually able to present a good face to the world. It's one of our ways of coping. Believe me, we are not always joking, happy-go-lucky clowns. We have our down times. Jack in particular is a worrier. I cope with that by taking a positive approach. We try to balance his negative times with my positive — sometimes we drive each other nuts, but we try to stay upbeat.

We also try very hard not to be critical of each other. My abilities with needles came to a head one night in a situation that could have gone two ways. We could have had a major disagreement that resulted in hurt feelings and a big fight. Or we could laugh. We chose to laugh. So picture this.

One snowy winter night Jack and I were driving home from Moncton. We were rushing to catch the ferry, so we couldn't stop. If we missed it we would surely be stuck for hours at the terminal waiting for the snowstorm to abate and the next boat to load and go to Prince Edward Island.

It was dark, snowing quite hard, and we were travelling at the maximum speed for the conditions. Jack suddenly realized he hadn't taken his insulin. He didn't want to stop and risk missing the boat, nor could he see the sides of the road well enough to pull onto the shoulder.

So he decided I should draw his insulin and inject it. Drawing the insulin into the needle was not that easy in a dark car on a bumpy road, but I did it.

"Okay," he coached, "pull my shirt up and give it into my stomach. That will be the easiest."

I was sweating. Just the thought of sticking that needle in his belly was freaking me out.

"Buck up," I told myself. "You can do this." Finally, I plucked up my courage, and jab, in went the needle. Right into his belly.

Bang! The car hit a bump. Out came the needle, before I could push the plunger. *Bang!* We hit another bump. Back in went the needle. Out, in. Out, in.

Finally, Jack grabbed my hand. "Wait! Not again," he grimaced. "Wait till the road smoothes."

Minutes later, his hand on mine, the needle went back in.

Now all I had to do was push the plunger thingy. Not easy, since I was restrained by a seatbelt and having a hard time reaching with both hands. Finally, with much jerking and moving of the needle I managed to inject the insulin. We just made it to the ferry and three hours later were pulling into our driveway.

The next day Jack had the biggest bruise on his belly! He made this big joke about me abusing him and made me promise to practise giving him injections. When things get tough today I'll sometimes give him "the look" and say, "Remember the belly needle." It always evokes a grin and a "Yes, Ma'am!"

Now, with that image in your mind, look at how far I have come. I'm proud of me and the way I have handled my husband's diabetes. I've learned so many things, *do* so many things I could never have managed before. I'm not perfect and never will be. I can be overly aggressive and bossy. I'm stubborn and a bit of a know-it-all at times. I'm overly protective, especially when someone or something is making life difficult for those I love and care about.

I want to remind all caregivers and supporters of diabetics that we are absolutely amazing in what we can do when we need to. If someone had asked me forty years ago if I could cope with things that are now just normal daily routine I would have vehemently said, "No way!"

Remember, I was a shy, introverted kid. When I was entering high school I was told to choose a course of study that would allow me to become self-sufficient. As my father put it, I should always be in a position to look after myself. To do that I had to be able to get a job. Since I had no thought of the professions — they were out of financial reach and I had no desire to be a doctor, lawyer, or accountant — I was basically presented with three options: nurse, teacher, or secretary.

Nurse was immediately out. I couldn't stand the thought of doing invasive things to people — the messy stuff, the blood. Heck, I fainted when the doctor gave me a needle. The thought of piercing skin (my own or someone else's) caused me to break out in a cold sweat.

Teacher? In Grade 9 I was living for the day when I could get out of school and certainly didn't aspire to work in one. That left secretary.

Oh, one of my cousins opted for hairdressing, but frankly I came from a family of non-touchers. Old school English, sort of standoffish folk. Although there was a mandatory bedtime peck of a kiss, it was a duty and not in any way casual contact.

Nope, no touchy-feely career for me. I improved when I married and certainly am huggy-touchy with my son and my husband. But anything invasive, like giving a needle — uh-uh, not me. Well, diabetes and aging have knocked that out of me. I still have a hard time with things that pierce the skin, but I can do it. And I do.

I handle the chores when I have to. I make phone calls, get argumentative, fight for Jack's rights for care and treatment. I no longer worry what people think of me when I request quick service in a restaurant or a fast appointment. Sometimes I feel like a banty hen, scratching the dirt back with my feet as I prepare to do battle, to take on whatever life throws at us.

I'm sure many of you are the same way. We deal with what we have to. We stretch ourselves and are amazed at what we can do. Any time you feel you just can't cope, look for some help — someone to talk to or to give you moral support. But rest assured that deep within yourself, whether you have diabetes or are concerned about a diabetic in your life, you do have what it takes.

That said, everyone has to be aware that they are dealing with another human being, and none of us are perfect. Frustrations can arise and can harm relationships.

MANIPULATION — HARD LESSON LEARNED

PK of Edmonton has long tried to be a true supporter for her diabetic friend. To find that she was being manipulated was a hard lesson, particularly because, as a caring individual, she had gone out of her way to help her both by providing special food for her diet and by waiting on her and giving her a chance to rest during her two-week visit.

In previous visits there had been a number of people around, so PK was never aware of the foods her friend was eating. Now, with family gone and PK and her husband following a healthy vegetarian diet, her friend did not have the same opportunity to sneak forbidden or limited foods.

That did not stop her from finding ways to pander to her cravings.

"She manipulated me to go and get her ice cream. She frightened us by saying her blood sugars were dangerously low. We offered her sugar, juice, and other things, but she insisted that only ice cream would work."

PK rushed to a store, worried about her friend. Soon the friend was gobbling down ice cream. And as a result she ended up ill from eating the sugary dessert. Worse, she destroyed a friendship that had been part of her life for years.

PK is very bitter at how she was manipulated and says it will forever change the supportive relationship she has tried to maintain for her friend.

THAT PARENT-TEEN THING

GM is a dad who is frustrated by his teenage son. He admits it is the "parent-teen thing" but says it is hard because he wants to "do" for his kid. He's frustrated because his son won't let him help. He resents that he's being shut out.

"It's difficult for adults when their children are diagnosed, no matter the age. But for parents of newly diagnosed teenagers it is particularly trying. My son is sixteen, was fifteen when diagnosed. I'm learning to keep my mouth shut and not say anything.

"A difficult situation for a dad. He does it all himself, is taking control. He's good. Good until he went to cadet camp. When he came home, he had the attitude he now knows everything. He's cheating a bit."

GM's son, he says, is not the kind of person you envision as a diabetic. He's slim, plays midget hockey, is active, and is president of the student council.

"I'm frustrated, but again, I'm just Dad, the village idiot. He's better with his mom. One seventeen-year-old we met blames it [his diabetes] on everything." GM's son doesn't do that. "He takes responsibility." However, he says, "He's starting to cheat now. He's feeling better and I've noticed him sliding."

His nephew was diagnosed at about the same time (two days before his first birthday). His wife compares notes with her sister, which has been a big help. "Especially because she had someone to talk to about it. It's really a family thing."

As frustrated as this dad is he is proud of his son. "He took it [his diagnosis] well. In hospital, his second day in intensive care, he was getting four needles a day. He said to the nurse, 'I guess I've got to learn to do this,' and he did. He's great that way."

"He's real good about the needles," GM says, relating how his son had interacted with a young child who was scared of having a shot. "He showed him it didn't hurt. He takes his needles himself and tests his blood as he's supposed to."

Still, he can't help but wonder why his son has diabetes. "I said to the doctor, 'What makes a young sixteen-year-old hockey player get this?' He said, 'If you can answer that, they will give you a million bucks.'"

CHAPTER 4
Working and Paying the Way

Probably the most difficult and dramatic influence that diabetes had on our lives was related to Jack's ability to work. Or perhaps I should say his determination to work. Many a lesser person would have been out on disability years before he opted for an early retirement.

It was only his intense management and control and his strength of will (read stubbornness) that kept him working.

When diagnosed as a diabetic Jack was holding down two jobs. He had his own business as a farrier, shoeing horses. He also had a mechanic's licence and had won a short-term contract position with Parks Canada. Thinking that job was just for six months he worked at the P.E.I. National Park by day and travelled from farm to farm on evenings and weekends tending the feet of horses. Both were physically challenging jobs.

When the job with Parks Canada became permanent he gave up shoeing horses. It had become too physically demanding — and his health was deteriorating. Going back to a regular eight-to-four job with scheduled lunch and breaks was certainly better for his health.

He was eventually promoted to a new position maintaining roads, trails, grounds, and all manner of things within the national park. He and his crew did a variety of tasks that ranged from convincing beavers to move their dams so that they didn't flood roadways to building bridges across tidal estuaries. They mowed grass along roadways that they also maintained, developed walking trails, floated an escaped boardwalk across a pond, cleared seaweed from a beach, buried dead whales, and in winter they cleared snow, plowed roads, spread sand and salt, and so on.

He loved the physical work and enjoyed the people he worked with but found the stress of being in a lower management position dealing with government bureaucracy trying at times.

As a diabetic his challenges were never knowing what level of physical activity he would be required to do on any given day; long, often unexpected hours, especially in winter when the intense cold was also a factor; and, most importantly, the stress.

In the mid-nineties his diabetes and overall health became worse. Work became a real struggle. From my perspective this was a terrible time. I worried constantly. Winters were the worst, especially if there was a snowstorm, freezing rain, or intense cold. Ever conscientious, Jack would head out as early as four o'clock in the morning to get to work. The roads were often unplowed and he had thirty kilometres to travel, most of it rural, and some of it uninhabited, with no help available if he needed it.

He would often not get home until late at night, as they worked to keep the plows on the road. I had no way of getting in touch with him. No communication. I spent many a night pacing the floor as the wind howled outside. I worried about him having no food. I worried about him having a low blood sugar reaction. I worried about him skidding off the road and freezing to death in a ditch. My list of worries was huge. When he did get home my relief would be tinged with anger that he had put me through all that anxiety. I was angry that he put a job above his own health and above me. Luckily, I couldn't stay angry at him for more than a minute or two.

Jack would stagger into the house, too tired to eat, sick with fatigue. Yet the next morning he would be off again in the wee hours. One of my biggest frustrations was his refusal to delay going to work until conditions improved, or to leave early when the weather got really bad.

The last winter Jack worked was the worst for me. I had reached the point of giving him an ultimatum. It's the job or me. I went along with his determination not to go out on disability, recognizing that it was a legitimate concern about someone else controlling his life mixed with pride and determination to stay independent. But I had reached the end of my rope. He was so ill by this point that many a day when he came home from work, even in the spring, he would collapse into his recliner chair, rousing himself only to eat, and then stagger to bed.

He agreed to put in for an early retirement and at age sixty left work. Realistically, Jack was able to continue working for as long as he did only because he had a great bunch of co-workers who helped him many, many times.

I know I dwell on winter a lot. Although I'm a person who copes well with most things, the worry factor related to Jack's working in the winter was huge. One of our greatest pleasures in the winter these days is enjoying an early morning coffee in our living room. Looking out the window we can see our neighbours shovelling their cars out as the sun rises. They have to get out to go to work.

We can wait till the plow goes by and the contractor who clears our driveway comes along. We are careful to keep lots of food and supplies on hand so we don't have to go anywhere. We have been known to call a cab or a friend to pick us up on his way rather than dig out the car.

Being self-employed with a home-based business I could always do those things, but now my pleasure is tripled because Jack is retired and can do them with me. Ahhhh, it's all part of our new quality of life.

I think working, holding down a job, is one of the greatest hurdles some diabetics can face. Diabetes and its effects can influence the ability to drive, the ability to see, the ability to do unexpected hard labour, the concentration, the reliability, even the ability to function at the same level all the time. Some jobs present so much stress that they are actually detrimental to a diabetic's health. In some jobs, with some employers, these factors make it difficult to continue.

Another factor is that diabetics sometimes require more sick time, so finding work can be hard. Co-workers need to be supportive and willing to become part of the support team. They need to be aware, to take action in the case of, for example, a low blood sugar reaction and understand that the occasional irritating behaviour might be the diabetes, not the person.

That said, I think a diabetic who has a good employer who understands the disease and works with the employee is in a truly great situation and will prove to be loyal and dedicated. A diabetic with a good job and a good working situation is a lucky person indeed.

WORKING SAFE

Work is such a hard topic to discuss in a book like this because there are so many variations of what people do to earn a living. In the course of writing this book the careers of people I talked to ranged from farmer to fisherman, from teacher to secretary, from executive to self-employed artisan, from paramedic to watchmaker. The variety was huge, but the factors affected by diabetes are the same. Some were very physical, labour-intensive jobs that put people alone or in dangerous situations. Others were desk jobs where the challenges were the sedentary day and the stress that came with their work.

This is just one of the reasons diabetes is such an individual disease. There is no model diabetic to emulate. Everyone has to realistically judge his or her own situation and how to deal with it. We can only offer a few tips and hints.

Whether you work outside the home all day or are engaged in more leisurely pursuits, keeping your blood glucose levels under control is vital. Here are some tips:

- Monitor glucose levels more often if you deviate from your normal routine and if you have had or will have more physical activity. A business lunch might be late or include food that you don't normally eat midday. Better to check than find yourself losing your edge because your sugars are high or low.
- Keep all diabetes care supplies with you, using a purse, carry-on bag, briefcase, backpack, or fanny pack. Use insulated bags with an ice pack when it is hot outside or even in a closed car on a cool but sunny day.
- Pack extra medication and blood glucose monitoring supplies when planning a trip away from home or if there is the slightest chance you may be delayed at work or sent on an unexpected trip. It helps you stay in control during unexpected delays. You should always have an extra battery for your glucose monitor and insulin pump.
- Carry a card or wear a bracelet identifying you as a person with diabetes.
- Always have a quickly absorbed sugar food (such as three glucose tablets, juice pack, or five or six pieces of hard candy) to treat a low blood glucose level.
- If you have to make business trips, ask your doctor for new prescriptions for all diabetes supplies and medications when travelling away from home in case you run out and need to get a refill.
- Time your insulin to the situation by discussing it with your doctor if need be.
- When eating away from home, wait until you see the food before injecting. This helps avoid low blood glucose levels when meals are delayed (i.e., in a restaurant, on a long car trip, at a friend's home, or in an airplane).

BUSINESS ABROAD

When leaving the country, go to http://www.idf.org for a list of International Diabetes Federation member associations. To find English-speaking doctors in foreign countries, go to http://www.iamat.org. You can always contact the Canadian Embassy if you need medical help away from home.

STRESS BE GONE

Anyone living with diabetes knows that stress, physical or emotional, affects blood sugars, although usually in different ways. Physical stress is usually caused by illness, injury, or even surgery. In Jack's case that usually causes blood sugars to rise and be harder to control. Emotional stress generally does the same thing but can work the opposite in some people. You need to learn to read your unique individual reactions by frequent testing.

Another thing I have noticed about stress is that it can trigger a period of not thinking right or even of not thinking at all. You can forget to do things that you normally do, like testing or keeping to your routine. You also act differently, eating or exercising more than normal. How often do we use feeling stressed or upset as an excuse to binge or eat something that usually never passes our lips? Or you might forget to take your meds, or even remember but say "To hell with it" and not take them purposely. It happens.

It is important for everyone to control stress, but I think it is more important for diabetics. If you have a high-stress job, you really might want to think about changing it for something less demanding. This is your health we are talking about.

Think about this: if you are in a high-stress job, and that stress sets off hormones and blood sugar reactions that impair your judgement, you might endanger other people. You might make bad decisions. You might endanger your own health. This is something to discuss with professionals. It helps them and you if you keep a logbook to record high-stress events and blood sugars taken at the time. You might see a pattern emerge. When Jack left his job he immediately noticed the effect of reduced stress. It wasn't just the job itself; it was as much the stress he put on himself to do it well. In his last years at work cutbacks meant many things he cared about were being neglected and services were lessened. That really bothered him. He would fret about it to the point where he was truly "stressed."

There are more ways to reduce stress than leaving your job, of course. Stress-management courses will help you learn to relax using special techniques. You can evaluate your own situation and perhaps institute changes to reduce stress. Even exercising, taking a walk, or enjoying a bit of down time will help reduce stress.

BEHIND THE WHEEL

In today's society most of us need a driver's licence to work. Whether we drive for a living or drive to get to our job, to meetings, or to make deliveries, the ability to drive is an important one. It is not to be taken for granted. Diabetics who drive for a living face special challenges.

Depending on where you live, what you do, and how you maintain control, there may be restrictions put on your licence. Low blood sugar reactions (hypoglycemia), vision loss, and other complications can influence the authorities to remove all or some driving privileges.

The unfortunate part of this situation is that many who are diagnosed with diabetes hide their condition for as long as they can and even refuse to seek proper medical treatment because they are afraid of losing their driving privileges, their job, and their lifestyle.

Take for instance a trucker who finds he has diabetes. What are the implications of that on driving into the United States? At the point of writing a long-haul trucker said diabetics were not able to haul across the border. What about salespeople calling on clients, or a cabbie — you get the idea.

There are several chronic complications of diabetes that may affect driving performance. We all think first of diabetic eye disease or incidents of hypoglycemia, but other things, such as nerve damage, heart disease, stroke, etc., can all affect this and other activities.

Unfortunately our system puts people into a self-protection mode when it comes to their eyesight and driving. Because of a fear of losing their independence and their driving privileges, some people refuse to seek proper medical care or to tell their physicians about vision problems.

The first indication that JP was to lose some of his driving privileges came when his eye specialist picked up his microphone and dictated a letter to the Department of Motor Vehicles recommending that restrictions be placed on his licence. It was a devastating blow. He had just retired, so it didn't affect his ability to work. However, if it had come a few weeks earlier it would have meant his job. As it was he had to give up his plan of working part-time driving heavy equipment, as well as the family's plan to travel in their RV.

This is a huge problem for people living in small towns or rural areas where there is no public transportation. It is a huge problem for people who rely on driving to get to work. So all too often they hide symptoms. Not something I would recommend, but something that is happening.

It is a tough call. Obviously governments are concerned with protecting the public and trying to prevent accidents. But at the same time, an overzealous doctor or official at the licensing bureau can affect the rest of someone's life.

So can a bad day. If you happen to be having a bad day when you get your eyes examined it can set in motion a scenario that can cause you much frustration and heartache if your physician is not willing to retest.

I must stress again that knowledge is power. So is determination to work for your rights. You can begin your quest for knowledge about driving as a diabetic at the Canadian Diabetes Association.

In assessing the suitability of people with diabetes to drive, medical evaluations are used to document any complications and to assess blood glucose (BG) control, including the frequency and severity of any hypoglycemic incidents. It is important to know that the level of licence you have can determine the degree of assessment. Obviously a commercial driver operating heavy equipment or driving an eighteen-wheeler is in a different situation than someone going to the store in the village for groceries.

The Canadian Diabetes Association's Guidelines for Diabetes and Private and Commercial Driving is available on its website at http://www.diabetes.ca/Section_About/aboutdriveguide.asp. The guidelines provide general recommendations for diabetes and driving as well as specific recommendations for private and commercial drivers. You will, of course, have to work with the regulations in your province of residence.

Much of the success that people will have in keeping their driving privileges depends on their own management. Every person must be assessed on an individual basis. That is your right.

It is your responsibility to take an active role in retaining your ability to drive. You must maintain your medical records by entering the results of your blood glucose monitoring in a logbook. That monitoring should be done with a blood glucose monitor that has been properly calibrated for the test strips you are currently using.

It is also your responsibility to ensure that you do not have hypoglycemic reactions while driving. That means you do everything possible to avoid a low blood sugar reaction by eating on time, eating the right things, taking appropriate medications when your should, and factoring in exercise and other things that influence your blood sugars. You must also recognize the signs that you are "going low" and be prepared to act immediately to correct the situation.

As a safety measure, and by law in some provinces, drivers should always test immediately before driving and at least every four hours while on the road.

A diabetic should never leave home without proper monitoring equipment, a supply of test strips, and a rapidly absorbable carbohydrate. We keep a bottle of a sports drink such as Gatorade in the car at all times.

RG, who manages his diabetes with diet and pills, travels a lot for his job. One of his management challenges is to remember to take enough of his medications to cover possible schedule changes.

"I can have two weeks' supply when I leave for a short trip to Toronto, then get an unexpected call to go across the country. From there I may have two or three deliveries before I make it home. Reality is I should always carry a month or more of my medication."

Of course driving is just one of hundreds of challenges for diabetics and work. Diabetics who have any element of danger in their job, such as working with industrial equipment or dangerous goods, are morally bound to take into consideration whether they are safe to be doing that job. They are also morally bound to manage their diabetes so that they are in top form!

No matter your occupation you need to consider the effect on your work — and its effect on you. When we met a watchmaker and listened to how concerned he is about his diabetes taking a toll on his vision it gave us insight into the many ways work can be affected.

INCENTIVE FOR "WATCHING HIMSELF"

DA of Nova Scotia has been on pills for five years and doesn't really feel the effects of his diabetes. The reason: he "watches himself." Something he says he has to do because of his work.

"I have a friend who is very bad. That influences me to watch myself," he says, stressing that it was hard when he found out he had diabetes. It "really hit home."

His work now presents his biggest challenge in controlling his diabetes. "I'm a watchmaker so any effect on my eyesight is important to me....My big problem is my job. I spend all my time doing watch repairs. I used to always be at pop and candy while I worked, would go through a pound of candy and two litres of pop a day."

To his credit, and because of the influence of his friend, he took control, building in little tricks that work for him.

"I stopped nibbling all the time and replaced it with an occasional piece of candy. Now I go to a machine in the mall. It spits out four or five pieces of candy, that's it. If I get on a real binge I buy a bag of candy, take out three or four pieces, and throw the rest out. I still have that feeling of buying it.

"If I'm biking I take two to four pieces with me. One secret is licorice pipes. I break off a little piece and it gives me a high amount of flavour. It's supposed to be good for my prostate as well. I found licorice pipes really good, then you get the real treat — the red beads [candy balls] at the end of the pipe."

Another way DA took control was to drop forty pounds. He wishes he could add more exercise to his routine, but although he says he sees little effect from his diabetes, he finds that work exhausts him. He says, "Most diabetics find when their job is done, they are done; burned out for the day," but that isn't the case for most people.

"If I could walk and exercise, I could do better, but I find that difficult to do. If I was to take one hour or two from my morning [to walk] I would be burned out and wouldn't be able to do my job. Put in a full day [of work] and it's the same. I'm too burned out to go out and walk.

"One thing I would like to see is a walking machine made so it is connected to a TV or computer. You would power it by walking. It would encourage people to stay and exercise; the television or computer game would provide the incentive to keep walking." It would, he says, enable people to get some exercise inside, "tied to a machine that provided something to do — not so boring while doing walking."

His recreation, motorcycling, burns energy, he says, but not the kind that counts as exercise for burning sugars for a diabetic. "It's not legwork."

His advice to pass along is something he notes from his friend who is so badly affected by his diabetes. It is for friends of diabetics.

"He goes house to house visiting friends, as many Maritimers do. Each one puts on a meal and is not doing something that suits a diabetic." That, he says, makes it hard. "Put a salad in. How many people buy a pie or cake or chips for when people come in. Instead ask if a person has diabetes and just have something they can eat."

SICK DAYS

It is a given. You will have sick days. Everyone has sick days. It is also a reality that illness, whether it's cold or flu, an infection, injury, or recovering from surgery, puts a diabetic's body under stress. The body has a method of fighting illness that involves releasing glucose. That can make your blood sugars rise, sometimes dangerously high.

For that reason every diabetic and her caregiver should make a sick day plan with the help of her doctor or diabetes educator. It should be written down so that the diabetic or her caregiver can easily follow it. Basically the plan should include increased testing of blood sugars, testing ketones, being careful to take medications on time and as prescribed, paying attention to food and fluid intake, and, most importantly, keeping track of what is going on.

If you are on insulin or oral medication you should have a scale or guideline for adjusting if need be (according to blood sugar and ketone values). If you don't understand or feel comfortable with checking your urine for ketones, please make an appointment with your diabetes educator to get up to date.

Your sick day plan should include directions for monitoring, medications, and guidelines for liquid and food consumption. You also need to know when to call your doctor. All of these things should be planned with a professional when you are well.

One thing I do know is that you should be careful about self-treating with over-the-counter medications, particularly those for sore throat, cough, and nasal congestion. Check with your physician or pharmacist before taking anything that is not prescribed. Many over-the-counter medications contain sugar or may not be compatible with drugs you are already taking.

GOOD NEWS FOR EMPLOYEES

One trend that is good news for diabetics is that a good number of employers have embraced the notion of investing in the health of their workforce.

"To the untrained eye, this approach could be seen as simply a nice perk for employees — a reward for their contributions to the organization," states a Canadian Diabetes Association supplement.

Called *Diabetes: Get Serious*, this print material included an article, "Investing in employees' health: Good business sense," which you might want to pass along to your employer.

The article says that while it is truly a perk for employees, the benefits of looking out for the long-term health of employees go much deeper for employers. It is good business to have healthy employees. It reduces costs caused by absenteeism, injury, and sluggish workers. It increases the quality and quantity of production when people are well and happy. There is also the fact that good help is hard to find, especially experienced help. Since most diabetics are Type 2 and usually over, say, forty-five, they are employees to value.

The focus of the association's piece is on prevention, but it does promote that businesses should provide the tools to ensure their employees are living a healthy lifestyle through a program called the Diabetes Workplace Wellness Program. Employers might well find it worth investigating.

Diabetics can be very valuable employees, especially if the employer is willing to work with them and understand what their realities and needs are. Let's face it. If you have diabetes and a good job you will be very aware of how valuable that is and give your all for your employer. Loyalty works both ways and can be a tremendous asset to all concerned.

Work, or a source of income, is one of the necessities of life. How we use the money we have is another matter. Most people I know who are battling diabetes find managing the financial aspect of living with diabetes as challenging as any other aspect of managing and controlling the disease.

A study, Diabetes Report Card 2001, again a project of the Canadian Diabetes Association, this time in partnership with l'Association Diabète Québec, uncovered some disturbing trends in the disparity of support and services available to people across Canada.

One, the "high cost and inequality of access to diabetes-related drugs and supplies," leads into the other topic of this chapter — money. The costs associated with being a diabetic are high. For most of us they will affect the quality of life for the rest of our lives. Of course if you are wealthy it won't affect you, but for those of us who fall into the middle- or lower-income class it's hard to see our so-called discretionary dollars being eaten up to maintain health. So what are those costs?

Drugs and medical costs obviously head the list. Medical treatment varies across the country, and there are hidden costs. In our case, for example, Prince Edward Island does not have a diabetes specialist, so we travel to Saint John, New Brunswick, for his appointments with his endocrinology and internal medicine specialist and his diabetes educator.

We would never, ever consider not going for our appointments — these folks gave Jack back a quality of life we thought was lost forever. However, I do want to point out that our provincial government does not offer any assistance to cover the costs of travel, even though it does not provide the services of an endocrinologist in province. The government covers the costs of treatment with the doctor and within the hospital, but not our travel. We cover those costs. It's a bit of a struggle, but we do it by juggling money.

What always concerns me is the number of people out there who can't do that — who can't find the money, who are being denied proper medical treatment because they are on pensions or have low income. Especially in cases where that low income is related to their inability to work because they have a disease like diabetes. It isn't right.

In the last few years we have had to travel to Halifax for both myself and Jack, as well as to Saint John. We do it and keep our receipts to claim the expenses on our income tax. But for many people, the reality is that they just can't afford it.

I once met a single mom who was working a full-time, low-end job, upgrading her education at night, and babysitting. All to make a better life for herself and her daughter. That little girl needed to go for kidney tests, but the cost of travel forced her to delay the trip. Just imagine being in a situation of having to delay medical treatment for a diabetic child because you couldn't afford it. She went for assistance but was denied. She was working.

Another diabetic, one of my husband's best friends, developed a serious disease or infection of the pancreas and was hospitalized several times in Halifax. The costs to his family of visiting him in the hospital were tremendous.

Knowing of these situations, and knowing the cost of such trips, led us, along with members of our motorcycle club, to set up a charitable fund offering assistance to people having to incur high travel costs to obtain medical tests or equipment. We know first-hand that having the stress of worrying about money added to the anxiety of a hospital visit is not a good thing.

Think about the costs. When Jack went on the insulin pump we made three trips to Saint John over several weeks. All involved overnight stays. When he started on the pump we were required to stay five nights in a hotel. Jack could have stayed in a facility for outpatients at a lesser cost, but I wouldn't have been allowed to stay with him there. Those first nights he was instructed to have someone there to help monitor and assist him, so we had to get a hotel room. I was in the room with him, and the representative from the pump supplier was in the room next door. She assisted us for the first two nights. In fact, she also assisted a mother and daughter who were doing a pump startup in an adjacent room.

Back to the costs. We spend about $100 per trip for gas, $39.10 for the toll on the bridge off the Island, and approximately $85 a night for the hotel. Then there is the cost of restaurant meals, parking at the hospital, etc. And, for me, there is the lost income. I'm self-employed. No work, no money.

Jack and I actually have it easy because I am self-employed. I can arrange to be away for a few days. Saint John is easily accessible to us — a five- to six-hour trip. We can drive and don't have to rely on public transportation.

Many do not have that accessibility to quality medical care. In fact Canadians are becoming increasingly nervous about the availability and quality of health care. And it's not just seniors. Baby boomers are nervous about how they are going to cope with their "golden years." The Canadian Labour Congress is quoted as saying that people are concerned about health care and not having enough to live on after retirement in a 2004 Canadian

Press Report out of Ottawa. Worrying about these things is an additional stress that people don't need in their lives.

IT MATTERS WHERE YOU LIVE

It matters where you live in Canada. Among the provinces and territories there are huge disparities in financial coverage of diabetes medications and devices, as well as access to financial assistance. The financial support available to Canadians managing their diabetes is inadequate. At the time of writing the Canadian Diabetes Association information said that, for example, insulin in Nova Scotia and New Brunswick is not covered. In P.E.I. insulin and ketone strips are partially covered, and steps taken in 2004 increased the amount the patient pays. In Nunavut both are entirely covered. In British Columbia, Alberta, Saskatchewan, and Manitoba coverage depends on your income. This situation is likely to have changed by the time this book is published, under the guise of health care reform. You need to check with each province and/or go to the Canadian Diabetes Association website under the Advocacy section.

These and other concerns mean that diabetics have to very carefully consider what they do, where they live, how they live, what they can afford, what they can do to save money. It all has to be carefully weighed. Considering a move to another province? You had better check out the availability of heath care first. What is covered? What is not? Can you access it without having to pay out a lot of money? Can you arrange for a doctor and have your records transferred before you go?

Truth is, there are a lot of things to consider beyond the cost of the moving van.

The lucky ones among us have good medical insurance, a drug plan, eye care, dental care, and foot care. But even then costs can be high and you have to work with, and within, the rules of your insurer.

TA of Prince Edward Island doesn't have medical insurance. She has two sons with diabetes. "The test strips alone cost on average $75 per month or $900 per year. The needles, syringes, etc., are an extra cost for Island diabetics too."

THE IMPORTANCE OF HEALTH INSURANCE

MS in New Brunswick wrote, "I am very fortunate to have a health care plan where my husband works. The cost to me is that I pay 20 percent and Blue Cross pays for the rest. My cost per month is about $65, not bad but I think that it could be better. The cost of the insulin is not bad, it is the test strips, which have a cost of almost a dollar per strip and they are something that gets thrown away. That can be very costly and that [testing] is one of the most important things that need to be done to keep your sugars in line. I test every day and sometimes twice a day.

"I can see why they're many people who do not test properly. That is crazy. You take a low-income, elderly, or one-income family trying to make ends meet as it is and they have to choose between this and feeding themselves, well I know what I would choose.

"It also costs a bit more on food because everything is a lot better if you prepare it yourself or buy fresh. Like vegetables and fruits alone can add up quickly if you need to have fresh in the middle of the winter. And you have to eat protein at every meal, so that may be an added cost also. You can't just have a slice of bread or a bowl of cereal, you need to make sure you have the proper amount of each group so your body can break it down properly.

"My doctor has been very good to me and wrote my prescription for a two-month supply at once so that I am only paying the one shot of $10 every two months, and that has saved some."

Speaking of insurance, it is one of the many barriers a diabetic faces. Diabetes can have ramifications on a person's eligibility for insurance on mortgage, disability, income, etc.

You may well find that restrictions are being placed on insurance that can affect your whole life and that of your family. For example, if you can't get insurance, can you buy a house, change your residence for something easier, smaller, closer to medical care? If you already have a home with insurance on the mortgage to protect your family, are you willing to give that up for a change of location? Last time we mortgaged we were told that Jack, as a diabetic, could not have the usual mortgage insurance against disability or death. The house and mortgage are in both our names, but when I applied for the insurance I was told that as the secondary person on the policy I had to make special application. The cost was prohibitive. Way, way above what we could afford. The only reason we got a mortgage was that the life insurance that we have had since we were first married would pay off the mortgage if one of us died.

So, be aware and be wary. Read policies very carefully to see if they have clauses about pre-existing conditions. Read the fine print to look for exclusions.

TRAVEL INSURANCE

Again, read the fine print. Make sure your travel insurance doesn't exclude you from benefits because of a pre-existing condition. Don't try to hide your diabetes and then later find out the policy is worthless. The Canadian Diabetes Association does have a travel health insurance program for members, so check it out.

COST SAVERS

Okay, let's tell it like it is. Diabetes is an expensive disease. No getting around it. But there are some things that people can do that are not all that expensive.

For instance, you could save quite a lot of money each month if you quit smoking. There is no cost related to getting the activity you need. The cost of low-dose Aspirin is four dollars a month, and a multivitamin will be about eight dollars a month.

There are of course drug costs and insulin supplies on top of that.

And those costs can be frightening. A quick tally of the expenses in our household showed that we pay out about $350 to $400 per month for drugs and supplies covered under our health care plan. Figure that out. We pay 20 percent. We are among the fortunate who have a medical plan that covers 80 percent of most drugs, insulin supplies, and dental, as well as eyeglasses every two years. Just imagine if we had to pay the whole shot! We simply could not do it. But even with our health care plan, we still have many expenses; the plan does not, for example, cover the frequent changes he needs in glasses.

Our provincial government recently increased the cost of insulin to and oral agents by $2 to $3 per unit (depending on whether you buy vials, cartidges or oral agents), estimating that most Islanders would have to pay only an extra $12 per month. Well, in our case they underestimated the number of cartridges used per month. I estimate this rise in insulin cost would impact our family by about $30 per month if our drug plan didn't pick up the extra cost. Doesn't sound like much, but add that onto our already frightening costs and it's easy to see why people are so upset about health care.

> **TIP**
>
> Take advantage of offers for free samples. For example, Accu-Chek recently included a card for a free test strip drum in one of its mailouts. You can also often get a tester free if you buy strips. If you don't use these offers yourself, then pass them along. They can save money. Disetronic, the makers of Jack's insulin pump, recently enclosed a coupon for free samples — we sent for them by return mail.

Many local offices of the Canadian Diabetes Association carry supplies such as meters, test strips, and dermatherapy products. It's worth investigating.

As I write this there is a report on the television news about the increasing numbers of seniors who have to go to the food bank to survive. Food banks in Moncton and Fredericton have seen the number of seniors using their services increase by six times since last year. The news report expressed deep concern about those with special dietary concerns such as diabetes. It takes work and planning to stay on your proper meal plan when your income does not increase in line with your ever-rising costs.

We certainly feel it in our household. I thank heavens that my work can be continued after I turn sixty-five, although there are concerns that I will lose it all in tax and clawbacks as the government continues its attack on seniors, those who are fighting health problems, and low-income individuals.

We do stock up on sale items at the grocery store, with a special eye out for frozen or canned fruits and vegetables that will keep. Right now my freezer is packed with blueberries, cranberries, corn niblets, and such, ready for winter. We buy organic beef from our local farmers' market, cutting quantity to allow us to have the better quality while remaining within our budget.

Every Monday Jack checks the flyers for specials. There have been drastic changes in how we shop. Being seniors who enjoy a morning coffee with friends at a coffee shop in a grocery store, we very seldom do a big shopping now. I don't buy bags of apples anymore. I buy one or two at a time. We buy fresh vegetables and meats to last two or three days at a time. This has virtually eliminated waste. Now I think portion size when shopping and don't overbuy. If I do get too much I freeze it, rather than increasing how much we eat or throwing anything away.

I have pulled out the old style of cooking that our grandmothers used. Cabbage, turnip, and carrots, the lower priced staples, are becoming more frequent in our diet.

We clip coupons for groceries and meals out. Like everyone else today we are frugal and careful. We will get by. Priority one in this household is, and will continue to be, maintaining health and quality of life.

It isn't just seniors who are feeling the pinch. Two gals who are coping with job layoffs, one of whom also has a severely ill husband, vented their frustrations. They have pride and want to be responsible but feel the help they need just isn't there.

THE FINANCIAL CHALLENGE

HB and NW have one thing in common. The two women can't afford to be diabetic. Both are on pills. Both have trying family situations to deal with. Both neglect themselves.

HB used to test every day after supper but says there is no support in her province for test strips. "Nothing seems to be done to help the diabetic maintain control and stay healthy. I have no money for test strips. Can't afford the food; the diet is expensive."

Her friend NW agrees but says they are okay because they don't feel too bad.

They both say the biggest challenge is the financial one. And certain things frustrate them.

"Test strips purchased from the diabetic association are more expensive than at the drugstore. If someone is in need — say, needs a few strips to do till payday — I thought they might help by providing them. But no."

CHAPTER 5
Living Life to the Fullest

A few short years ago Jack lost his younger sister to lung cancer. A year later, almost to the day, he lost his younger brother to the same disease. They were the youngest in a family of four, and both could have been poster people for good health. George was ex-military without an ounce of fat evident on his body. Sue was always physically active and slender. Both died within six months of being diagnosed and were too ill to travel or do much of anything for their last months. Both were in their early fifties.

All of their lives Jack's sister and her husband had put off doing things with the idea of really enjoying their retirement. I will never forget the frustration, sorrow, and anger at fate that our brother-in-law expressed after her funeral. Here he was, better off financially than they had ever been, but without his soulmate to enjoy the rest of his life with.

That more than anything brought home to us the importance of living life to the fullest while you can. Aside from the fact that Jack has diabetes, we are aging. I have a great fear of finding myself in the position of my brother-in-law, filled with regret for things put on hold.

We are very aware that Jack has a limited time when he will be able to travel the way we would like to. His eyesight is a concern — we don't know how long he will be able to drive and to see the things we want to see. We notice things that mean revising our ambitions as far as travel goes.

This year, for example, he sold his BMW touring motorcycle. He loved his bike but no longer had the leg strength he needed to ride it. His dream had long been to go across Canada on the motorcycle. He could never do it when he was younger. He never had the vacation time or the money. Now, the only way he could have his cross-Canada odyssey is if a) he gets a smaller, lighter bike that is closer to the ground, and b) we have a sudden influx of cash. Unless we win the lottery it ain't gonna happen.

Selling the bike was very difficult. We both love motorcycling and hated to let it go. We have a new dream now of getting a small RV. Everyone thinks we're nuts, with the cost of the RV, the cost of fuel, and the fact that I may be the only one able to drive it. But consider our reasoning.

We love the outdoors, camping, and travelling, and the RV would make it feasible. We would have our own space. A home to go to. Over the past few years I have been changing my work so that I can do it from anywhere. I can write as we travel.

I have travelled a lot in the course of my work and find the most tiring aspect to be lugging luggage in and out of hotels. Living out of a suitcase is not the best for a packrat like me!

We find the hardest things about travel are keeping Jack on his own food and routine and getting a good rest. He doesn't sleep well on any given night, moving from the bed to his recliner virtually every night. I always laugh and warn visitors that he "sleeps around." It is a good laugh, but it's also the reality. I figure having our own bed and kitchen facilities would be well worth the cost. Even if we park in someone's driveway and visit them all day, he would have his place to rest in comfort and I would have my office.

The reality is that diabetics have down days. We accept them as "crash days," when Jack is going to feel miserable and not want to do much more than veg out. In an RV we can just pull over and stay put, in comfort, until he is ready to move on.

We have family and friends scattered across the country, people we want to see and spend time with. Jack's mother, sister-in-law, and nephew are in Victoria, British Columbia. Our son and his wife are in Vancouver. Jack's remaining sister and her family are in Edmonton. My mother and family are in southern Ontario. We have friends in almost every province.

Living life to the fullest is not limited to travel. Jack had long wanted to play golf, but he never had the time, energy, or money to enjoy it. Now that he is retired and has the improved health brought about by his insulin pump we budget for his membership so that he can play all summer long. It isn't easy to come up with that money. In fact we have cashed in RSPs to pay for his membership and a spring golfing vacation in Ontario. But it's worth it.

The daily exercise and the fact that he has a group of friends and an activity that make his retirement a pleasure make the expenditure a good one. In the winter he shifts over to skating and attending hockey games, but we are striving for the day when we can take golfing vacations in the winter. Right now I'm still working, so our living-life-to-the-fullest options are influenced by my schedule. It won't be much longer, though, before I'm out there with him.

In the meantime, we attempt to live life to the fullest in every way we can — even if that happens to be coffee at the grocery store with our friends.

What do we mean by living life to the fullest? It varies from person to person and from day to day, but basically I would say it's taking out those dreams, those things you've always said you want to do, and rethinking them. If you really want to do those things, then put the steps in motion and go for it.

Like everyone, as we age our health and our ability to do things is changing. Diabetes makes us more aware of that life clock ticking as symptoms present themselves. If there is one thing to consider it is this: do you want to wake up one day filled with regret at what you've missed? Do you want to let your good days drift on by without making the best of them?

You will benefit in so many ways from living life to the fullest. The increased enjoyment of life and activity level will do you nothing but good.

There are so many wonderful things out there that people enjoy doing. I can't possibly cover them all in this chapter, and this book is sort of about us, our friends and acquaintances, our lives, so I'm going to focus on an activity that we enjoy — travelling. We also enjoy golf, motorcycling, walking nature trails, and so on. But for many of us travel is part and parcel of what we love to do. More and more often, it is also required for our work.

I'm sure we could write just as much about anything you do. In the meantime, take these things we enjoy as examples of how you can enjoy the things that appeal to you.

Every year our motorcycle club here in Prince Edward Island puts on a rally over Labour Day weekend. The event attracts almost five hundred motorcycle touring enthusiasts from Canada and the U.S.A. As a volunteer I was manning a table in the main hall, selling fifty-fifty tickets to raise money for our charity. Since I was working on this book I put up a sign looking for diabetics to interview.

At first it seemed that most of the people coming up were men, obviously over fifty and more obviously overweight. But as we continued talking to people the pendulum swung. More and more women came forward. None of them were grossly over-weight. It was an interesting mix. The stories told by several of the people we talked to are in this book. What was really amazing was the fact that nearly 10 percent of the attendance came forward as either a diabetic or as someone living with diabetes in one way or another. That was scary!

What was impressive was the willingness of these folks to share their experiences and the ways that they were striving to manage their diabetes so that they can continue to enjoy an activity they love — touring on their motorcycles.

REGULATED RIDING

JS and his wife, MS, had travelled more than two thousand kilometres from the Catskills in New York State on a Gold Wing to attend the rally. JS, a friendly guy, has a big belly. A stroke gives a sleepy look to his right eye and, as he says, his grin only works on one side of his mouth. JS controls his diabetes with pills and is very aware that when he is riding, he has to be right on.

"Two big things you've got to remember: if you don't keep regulated you don't feel good. You pass out," he said, smiling. "Not a good thing."

He has numerous ailments and problems related to his heart, blood pressure, and arthritis, and he has a blind spot in one eye. "And I don't heal worth crap," he added.

"Just gotta be careful. A friend was helping me push my bike back four years ago. I said let me do it myself, but he insisted. It came back and hit my leg. Broke my toenail — turned it black and blue. It's still not gone four years later. You've gotta be careful, keep it regulated."

Diabetes runs in his family. "My mother has it. Our daughter got it when she was pregnant with her second child and has never gotten rid of it. She's on two needles a day."

For all his talk about regulating, JS admits he is not the best at testing his blood sugars. "I get sick of fingers being sore and give up. I know I'm gonna see the day when I have to test more. I'm sixty years old. If I start having trouble I'll test."

JS admitted to being more careful with his management when he was on the road than when he stopped for a few days like the time spent at the weekend rally. After spying him eating an ice cream cone I asked him about his challenges.

"I love ice cream. My biggest challenge is binge eating. You have to live. I find it so hard to watch what I'm eating."

So how does he stay healthy enough to drive a motorcycle, with his wife on board and saddlebags loaded? He works at it, but he is the first to admit he needs help. He and his wife act as a management team.

"If I work I feel better. I keep active. The minute you stop doing things you're done. My wife is my saviour. My number one supporter." A borderline diabetic herself, she is his watchdog.

"I make sure he takes his pills every day," she butts in. "He hates it, but I'll get after him to at least eat a slice of toast and take his pills in the morning. If not he forgets. He hates taking pills, says he takes so many."

Even so, she keeps him on track. "As long as he's taking the pills he's fine. If not he starts feeling sick right away. He calls every day at noon, and I'll ask, 'Did you take them yet?' Sometimes he'll say no but says he will as soon as we get off the phone. I will call again later and ask again. I can tell by the way he answers that he hasn't taken them. He'll promise to take them as soon as he gets off the phone."

JS, who works as an emergency medical technician, and MS wander away to talk to friends, but soon JS is back. He has something he needs to say. He sits down and starts talking of a friend who will never ride his motorcycle again. He lost his leg, and finally his life, to diabetes. It affected JS deeply.

"I'm fanatical about anything happening to my legs. The pad of one foot is numb now. I probably wouldn't know if I got a sore, so my wife checks my feet all the time. I'm an EMT. I know how critical this can be."

Yet JS isn't perfect, and some of the signs are not encouraging. "I'm so exhausted and I haven't done anything."

Now they stay in a motel, instead of on site, and miss some of the activities at the rally so that he can rest. I suspect he needs to re-evaluate with his physician if he wants to be riding his motorcycle four thousand kilometres again next summer.

TRAVEL TAKES SMARTS

Travel affects your routine, whether it is a short or a long trip. It exposes you to different, hard-to-count foods. You need to stay alert and work to stay in control. Whether travelling for business, personal affairs, or a vacation, you need to plan and prepare ahead so that you can have a worry-free, enjoyable trip. We, for example, now plan all of our trips to exclude flying.

The year Jack got that magic combination of age and years worked that made him eligible to collect his pension also happened to be the year of his mother's eightieth birthday. She'd had a rough couple of years. Jack's stepfather had died in late winter — while they were on vacation in Florida. We all rushed to Ontario to help his mom get through the trauma and talked to her about moving to be near one of her children. She opted for the milder climate of Victoria, B.C., and moved there in July, purchasing a small house just a couple of blocks from Jack's brother. Just a few months later, in December, George died of lung cancer.

For years the family had joked that George and their mom, both avid smokers and beer drinkers, would celebrate her eightieth birthday by throwing a big party. It seemed right that we go for the occasion, especially since George was gone. It was also our first vacation together in more than a decade. We boarded the plane to Vancouver with great anticipation. We knew Jack would need some down time to get over the flight and the four-hour time difference, so we scheduled a few days R & R before heading over to Victoria to be the "surprise" at his mom's party.

The party and visit were great, but Jack seemed brittle. I could sense that he was having to work at being cheerful and enjoying things. By week three I knew he was going on adrenalin, stubbornness, and sheer willpower. The last few days he was in trudge mode.

I can always tell when he's heading for a setback. He tries to be up, active, and cheerful, but he gets a grey pallor to his skin. He shuffles his feet instead of stepping; his mouth gets tight, lips thin. He has to concentrate more on what he is doing. He also gets super cheerful, almost exuberant, for short periods of time but then swings the other way and gets all quiet. I liken it to an engine running with a partially blocked fuel line.

So during this trip he worked to present a cheerful face and I worried. The day we boarded the plane home I was swinging between sorrow to be leaving, relief that I was going to get him home to our own medical support, and apprehension about the flight.

Halfway across Canada I knew we were in trouble. He was grey, his breathing laboured. We kept a close eye on his blood sugars. He slept a lot. I watched him. Thankfully we live close to the airport so I got him home and into bed before he collapsed. He was down and out for over two weeks. This episode led to a fast deterioration of Jack's vision described elsewhere in the book. It was over a month before he started getting back to feeling decent.

The reality is that Jack is a brittle diabetic and just plain cannot fly. Crossing four time zones (especially travelling west to east), getting off schedule, the pressure, the lack of oxygen in the plane, and the stress of changing planes (travelling coast to coast can result in a nightmare of rushing and running to catch connecting flights in Toronto and has me vowing never to fly that way again) is just too much for his system. Our doctor has been very firm in stating that he should not fly — and this episode really brought it home to us.

We travel. But now we plan it to be the least stressful that it can be. We go by car or train, and that way we both enjoy ourselves.

BEFORE YOU GO

There is a saying that the planning is half of the fun, so make sure you get your full quotient of fun from travelling by spending lots of time working out the details. Here are a few tips that will help get you started.

- When booking your ticket ask your travel agent to schedule in a way that suits your routine and also order any special diabetic meals. Consider alternatives to air travel. Trains are great! Incidentally, I recommend using a travel agent. If anything does go wrong, if there is illness or an "incident," a call to your travel agent will help resolve things. A friend was in Indonesia, heading home to Prince Edward Island, when 9/11 put world airlines in a frenzy. He called his travel agent, who made the arrangements to get him back on Canadian soil and safe.

- Make an appointment with your physician for several weeks before you travel. Some countries require a "proof of need" statement that includes a list of health problems and major illnesses and medications (both prescription and non-prescription). Did you know that the United States sometimes requires a copy of your prescription and proper identification on the pharmacy label for drugs? Get the proper documentation detailing your condition and any special things medical caregivers and security or customs officials might need to know, as well as a list of all medications you are taking. This is really important if you are leaving the country. Note that travelling with syringes or needles without appropriate medical documentation can lead to serious trouble with authorities in some countries.

- If you have to cross time zones ask your doctor for help in adjusting your routine, which is especially important if you use insulin. This is vital if you cross several time zones in a short time (e.g., when flying) because your routine gets thrown out the window. We all know that being in control of timing and routine is the key to good health. Because Jack has trouble adjusting to crossing several time zones, we always plan two days of quiet time before beginning family visits or travel once we reach our destination.

- Visit your pharmacy several weeks ahead. Tell them you will be travelling and will need extra prescriptions. If you will be gone for a long time they may not have enough stock on hand to fill your order. As well, many insurance companies will pay for only a month's supply at a time, so if they do direct billing you may need to make special arrangements. If you submit your receipts for reimbursement from an insurance company ask them how to handle buying a larger than usual supply. Again, you can save yourself a hassle by planning and acting ahead.

- Get your pharmacy to give you a letter detailing all of your medications, both prescription and non-prescription, just in case you need to replace any. This should include the doses you are taking and the drug's name and DIN (drug identification number).
- Wear a bracelet or necklace identifying you as a diabetic and carry an up-to-date medical card in your wallet.
- Get in the habit of journalling. Jack uses a small appointment book as well as his logbook. He notes when he should change the site for his pump. When we travel I document things such as what we eat, where, and when. We document any blips or bad days. The thing about journalling is that it makes you more aware of what you are doing and makes it a little harder to slide into bad habits. It also documents what you have been doing, which is invaluable if you get into trouble.

It is vital to research the requirements of the country you will be visiting, countries you will pass through, and Canada. Start with these websites:

- Health Canada Travel Medicine Program: http://www.hc-sc.gc.ca/pphb-dgspsp/tmp-pmv
- World Health Organization International Travel and Health: http://www.who.int/ith/
- Canadian Society for International Health listing of travel medical clinics in Canada: shttp://www.csih.org/index.html
- U.S. Department of Health and Human Services, Travelers' Health, Centers for Disease Control and Prevention: http://www.cdc.gov/travel/

If you are in business, check with government offices that deal with exporting and international affairs. They publish handy little information books about many countries.

You can also obtain information from embassies or tourism offices of various countries. Your travel agent should be able to help you sort it out.

INSURANCE

As a diabetic you may find it difficult to get travel insurance. This is true especially if you are insulin dependent or travelling to an "exotic" location, but even travel insurance for the U.S. is expensive and hard to get.

It is important to review your insurance situation *now*. If you have an existing policy that covers your travel, whether through employment, a credit card, or other program, be sure that you don't let it lapse. If you don't have anything that you can continue start shopping. The Canadian Diabetes Association has an insurance plan for members. Check it out.

Research well and always read the fine print. If it says pre-existing conditions may not be covered be very careful before you sign on the dotted line. Ask questions and get the answers in writing.

Read the fine print before paying for any insurance. When my father-in-law died in Florida his insurer indicated they would not pay his hospital or ambulance bills because my mother-in-law dialled 911 before she called them. The insurer dictated which hospitals they could use in an emergency.

If you are communicating with insurance companies via email print off and keep the correspondence. If you are communicating by telephone record it, or at least take notes that you file with the date, name of the person you talked to, and time of the call.

It might sound like overkill, but a little forethought now can save much hassle and possibly money down the road.

INSURED AND READY

We all know it's important to carry insurance documents when we travel, but anyone with insurance for drugs or supplies is wise to carry a couple of submission or claim sheets for reimbursement of the costs of drugs. If you do happen to have to get a prescription filled on vacation you will probably have to pay for it up front. If you have your claim forms with you then you can mail them in immediately. Our payments go into our bank automatically, another good idea if you are travelling for any length of time.

AIR TRAVEL

Pack your own meal with a focus on non-perishable, easily transportable food items: a cheese sandwich, an apple, a banana, veggie sticks, low-fat yogurt, juice, crackers, or cookies. If you don't need it, it's not a big thing. If you do need it, it's a godsend. There are so many reasons to be in control of what and when you eat on an airplane: delayed flights, slow food service, an unsuitable airline meal, times that don't suit your schedule.

Although some airlines offer diabetic meals, they require advance notice, often the meals don't arrive, and frankly the people who make them sometimes have a pretty strange idea of what a diabetic can or needs to eat.

Keep all medications and special supplies with you. Don't ever assume that your luggage will arrive when you do.

If you are insulin dependent and need to carry syringes you had better have a doctor's letter stating that. We also get a print-out from our pharmacist. Keep all medications, including syringes, in their original packaging so that they are easily identified. Just in case they are confiscated, put an extra supply of syringes in your luggage. If they try to take your syringes from you insist that the needles you will need during the trip be held by airline cabin staff until you need them.

Crossing time zones? You must be prepared to gradually adjust your routine. Make sure you have planned this ahead and then pay attention to the timing of both meals and medication.

Move as much as you can. Start in the airport. Don't just sit in those plastic seats like a blimp: get up, walk, and stretch. Once in your seat do periodic stretches, ankle twirls, neck rotations, even knee raises. Get up when it is safe to do so and walk up and down the aisles to get your circulation going. Bend over and touch your toes. Do some side bends. Don't worry about other people watching you; there are so many fitness buffs today that you will fit in.

Dress for comfort and good health. Don't wear restrictive clothing. You need to be able to move around. Wear sensible walking shoes.

CRUISES AND TOURS

Cruising? Get your travel agent to check for cruise lines that offer diabetic or specialized meals and have flexible of mealtimes. Also ask the agent about any related costs for these services and about the medical personnel who will be on board.

Tour groups present a challenge because their schedule may not coincide with yours and many meals are set in advance. There is no choice. Before you book any tour, ask about how your needs for proper meals served on time can be met. Be prepared to take along your own food, to eat on a bus or on the go if need be, and forgo the meal that goes with the tour.

Again, move around when you can. I met a group from a cruise ship in the food court of our local mall. One lady was obviously not well. Her friends knew she was diabetic — and, as one put it, a stubborn old fool — so they had decided to just dump her in the food court to fend for herself because she spoiled all of their land excursions. "Maybe she'll learn to walk a bit and eat properly if we don't cater to her," said one elderly gentleman.

IN THE HOTEL

Okay, how easy is it to flop on the bed and veg out in front of the TV? Don't forget that you need to keep your exercise routine. Not easy if you have been sitting all day as you travel. Check out the fitness room or the pool. Ask the front desk staff for maps and directions to safe places to walk.

GROUP PLANNING

Each year a family gets together in Truro, Nova Scotia, a mid-point location for Mom, sisters, brother, and their families, who are scattered throughout the region. A stay in a hotel with a great pool has become a traditional vacation weekend. But, this year, with Mom now coping with diabetes, DG, the main member of her mother's management team, realized that the rest of the family, who had not been through any educational training concerning their mom's diabetes, were not considering her needs.

"At 8:00 p.m., we hadn't had supper yet. I finally had to say to them, 'Look, Mother needs to eat.' They just don't get it," says DG. She knew her mother would never make an issue of the late meal.

It is a fact of life that if one of a group is diabetic, then everyone in the group needs to just rethink a little, especially when away from home. After all, a healthy group is a happy group, and eating on time is a small price to pay for happiness.

On the earlier mentioned trip to Vancouver, Jack and I learned very valuable lessons about handling insulin. We rented a car and did a bit of exploring on Vancouver Island. The weather was glorious — and hot. He had his insulin and drugs in a carry bag that we always kept near us — leaving it in the car when we went to hike, explore, or shop. After a few days he began to feel sick. His blood sugars were all out of whack. No matter how he adjusted his insulin, it didn't help.

PACKING LIST

The following items should be kept with you at all times when travelling. Do not put them in checked luggage:

- a doctor's letter detailing your medications and any special treatment
- all required medications in their original containers
- travel and medical insurance documents

Then, bingo, it hit us. We were actually talking about cold drinks and the regret that we didn't have a cooler filled with ice when the light went on. We had unintentionally cooked his insulin. Off we went to the drugstore. They agreed that the heat had probably affected it, called our own drugstore back in P.E.I., and in no time Jack had not only new insulin but also a Styrofoam cooler, some ice, and a plastic container to keep the insulin in. The cooler cost $1.99. The insulin, $180.

A year later we set out to drive to Ontario. Between Moncton and Fredericton Jack asked me if I would get a vial of insulin out of the cooler to warm. He would soon need to put a new vial in his pump. No insulin. He asked if I had put his insulin in the cooler.

"Me, no! You said not to do anything with your 'stuff,' that you would pack it."

He didn't because we had broken our usual routine, which sees Jack pack the cooler. This time I put the food in but didn't think of his insulin. So, we hauled off the highway in Fredericton and again had to purchase it on the road. This time it cost $190.

Several important lessons learned. Always carry forms to submit receipts to our insurance company. In both cases we had to wait several weeks after returning home to get reimbursed for an expenditure we didn't need while on vacation. Now we carry forms and payment is set up to go automatically into our savings account.

And we always carry insulin in an insulated bag or cooler. Oh, and we double-check that we have all medications and supplies actually in the car.

KEEP YOUR COOL

It is very important to look after your insulin when you travel.

You need to keep your insulin cool. If flying, small totes or insulated bags are ideal, but many of us rent cars at our destinations and travel in hot weather. Then you need a little more cool power. Cheap Styrofoam coolers can be purchased almost anywhere. Rather than relying on hotel/motel ice cubes (which melt fast) get several ice packs, or fill small water bottles three-quarters full, squeeze to get a bit of the air out, and put the caps on tight. The squeezing makes room for expansion when the water freezes. Explain that you are carrying insulin that has to be kept cool and any hotel or motel will pop half of your ice packs in the freezer overnight.

If you are taking a driving holiday an electric cooler is great. Just make sure that it stays on the cool setting, not the hot one.

GENERAL COMMON SENSE

Travelling, whether it's a day trip close to home or an extended vacation, will always be the most successful if you use a little bit of common sense along the way.

- Always carry a snack pack that includes non-perishable snacks and a quick-acting form of glucose (tablets, candy, juice).
- Strive for a balanced diet away from home.
- Journal what you eat, when you take medications, etc. The act of writing it down becomes habit and serves as a reminder. It keeps you on track and helps you identify what works for you and what doesn't. Being able to trace back can be very helpful.
- You don't have to eat everything put in front of you, especially if the timing is wrong. Share your meal or ask to have it packed to go. Order smaller portions.
- Whether you travel by plane, train, or automobile, you need to exercise. It keeps you healthier and burns some of those sugars. Stretches in your seat, walks up the aisle, striding around an airport or station — any movement is better than none.

TIMING IS LIFE

Nova Scotian SM, who takes three pills a day to control her diabetes, says timing is her life.

"Through the summer it's hard. I get out of routine with the kids home. It's a challenge trying to stay on my diet. Travelling is hard if we can't find a place to stop and get something to eat. I carry food now more than I used to."

Diabetes is part of life for SM but has presented challenges for her family. She has a real understanding of what her boys go through because she experienced the same thing with her own father. He had it "really bad," as did her grandmother and older sisters. In fact knowledge of their diabetes led her to go to get tested for it at the doctor's.

"My husband is really helpful, but the boys are scared I'm going to die. They won't let me eat things like chips. They say, 'I'm not going to kill you.' It can be scary, what the boys feel."

That knowledge gives her the impetus to work to keep good control.

"My father just didn't care. We worried about him till the day he passed. I lived with a diabetic and have a better understanding of how it affects family."

Diet and exercise are part of how she works to maintain good control. She has gone from a size twenty-four to a sixteen, so feels she is "not doing too bad."

"The foods that are hard for me? Pastas. I love them, but pasta makes me shoot right up. I feel like I'm groggy. Use moderation and you do pretty well.

"I go to Curves [a women's fitness centre] and feel ten times better for getting active.

"I feel that just coping is a major thing. Every so often it hits me and I go off on a crying spell.

"Mood swings? Oh yeah, and my family knows. If I'm really trying and get frustrated or upset they stay away. They know. They just leave."

IT'S A DOGGONE GOOD THING

Hard to get motivated? Consider a pooch. No one can be unaware of how valuable service and assistance dogs are becoming in our society. I'm sure many of you know about the dogs that can detect the onset of seizures or even sense cancer. One television program profiled a dog that actually senses when its owner is close to having a low blood sugar reaction. These are important skills that require intense training.

Most of us are not likely to have the services of these highly skilled pooch detectives. But we are in a position where we can benefit from the love and motivation that a dog can bring into our lives.

I've long felt that our miniature schnauzer, Tipsy, plays a really important role in Jack's health as well as my own. She cheers us, cajoles us into walking, and has just brought us smiles and joy right from the day we got her. She loves us unconditionally. She puts us to bed at night and gets us up and going in the morning.

A few weeks ago she proved another value a dog can bring into life. Jack had taken her for a long walk on a nature trail. It was a beautiful fall day and he went further than usual. He began to feel "off" and recognized the signs that he might be going low. About halfway back to the car Jack knew he was in trouble. He was starting to stumble and was feeling disoriented.

"I knew if I sat down, or went down, I would never get up, so I put Tipsy on her lead and told her to take me to the car. She did. She must have sensed I was in trouble because she just went out to the end of the lead and motored back instead of her usual sniff and explore saunter.

"There is a wooden bridge just before where we park. I vaguely remember wanting to sit there, wanting to lean on the railings. She kept tugging and got me to the car. I fell into the back seat. I knew my Gatorade was there and drank the whole bottle. It took a good ten minutes before I could sit up. She sat there with me the whole time. I felt safer, and she was something to focus on that kept me from giving in to the reaction out in the boonies."

Jack had made two mistakes that day. His miscounted his meal and took too much insulin as a result. He went for a walk with no source of sugar in his pocket. He always has a sports drink in the car and glucose tablets and hard candy in his fanny pack. But that was in the car instead of on his hip.

This incident was a wake-up for us. We have since got him a small voice-activated cell phone that he *will* carry. He *will* also double-check his pockets for a sugar source before heading out on the trails.

CHECK YOUR CODES

"The doctor wanted me to a test four times a day. I was all over the place: 3.0, 10.0, 13.0. I was getting worried. Then I happened to look at the code. I'd forgotten to change it with the new vial of test strips."

— JG

You must calibrate your meter!

The one problem with walking the dog for exercise is their habit of stopping to sniff. Remember that brisk walking is what you need. Those stops don't mean you should just stand there. Flex your muscles, move around, and get pup back on track.

CHAPTER 6

Interpret and Understand

In the late 1990s Jack's health was deteriorating alarmingly.
He felt out of control although he worked very hard at eating
properly, taking his medications as prescribed, and doing
everything he was told to do. He felt desperate and was con-
vinced he would not survive for much longer. He had no life.
If he wasn't working or sleeping he was most likely in his
recliner watching television. Most days he just didn't have the
energy to add much else to his routine. He was too ill. The
days that he did feel good were devoted to household chores,
keeping the cars in order, squeezing in a bit of living.

So there he was watching golf on television. At the end of
a tournament the announcer interviewed a golfer who had
been absent from the pro circuit for a number of years. He
was noteworthy because of his remarkable comeback. I did-
n't see the interview, but when Jack told me about it he was
optimistic and had a feeling of hope for the first time in a
long time.

The golfer had an insulin pump. He was very eloquent
about how going on the pump had changed his life so much he
was able to return to professional golf. Jack began to look for
more information on the pump. He asked our family doctor, but

he was unfamiliar with them. The Diabetes Association dismissed them as too expensive.

He kept asking. Our doctor came through, telling us about an individual in Prince Edward Island who had a pump. We never met him, but our doctor did. I remember his amazement over seeing this fellow eating cherry pie and ice cream in a restaurant. Dr. Carruthers, our family doctor, arranged a referral to Saint John Regional Hospital in New Brunswick, where a specialist would evaluate Jack to determine whether he was a good candidate for pumping. Things were set in motion.

We were immediately impressed with the people and facilities at Saint John Regional Hospital. The first doctor we saw assessed Jack's medical history and stunned us when he said he did not feel Jack's condition warranted his going on a pump, so he would not recommend it. But, he continued, the final decision would rest with Dr. John Dornan.

Long minutes later Dr. Dornan came into the room. He checked the information over and then asked Jack why he felt the pump was important. His A1Cs were good. He seemed to be in control of his sugars.

Jack told him the realities of his life. He had heart and kidney problems and experienced persistent exhaustion. He had lost a great deal of his vision. We never got a vacation because he always had to use his vacation days for sick time. He felt he had no life. In fact, at that point he felt like he did not have long to live.

Dr. Dornan listened intently, checked a few things, and then turned to the other doctor, and in his quiet but authoritative voice said, "I'm sorry, I have to disagree with you. I feel Jack is an excellent candidate for pump therapy."

Jack squeezed my hand so tightly I almost snatched it away. Almost. One look at the relief in his eyes had me squeezing right back. Dr. Dornan briefly detailed how the process would proceed. We needed to get our insurance coverage and monies lined up, obtain an insulin pump, get comfortable with handling the pump, learn how to properly count carbohydrates, and get ourselves educated to a new way of life. Then we could return for pump startup. It was a daunting list, but doable.

We had been researching pumps. Not easy. There was very little information available in Prince Edward Island. I didn't feel right turning to the Internet because we needed something within our region. Neither Jack nor I felt comfortable not dealing with a person. This was his life we were talking about, and we felt we needed a person to guide us, to answer our questions, and to hold our hands through a tense time.

It was tense for several reasons. We felt like we were bucking our provincial system. Our family physician backed us all the way, but we were going into uncharted waters. Were we crazy insisting on this thing that no one else seemed to even acknowledge? Could we do it? The implication from many was that it would be too complex, too difficult for Jack to manage with his deteriorating eyesight. Was it worth the time? Could we afford the expenses, not just for the pump but also for the travel to Saint John and accommodations while there?

Now I would do a "Google" search as a starting point to get local contacts and some basic knowledge. I would go beyond our local chapter of the Diabetes Association for basic knowledge. Today they are better informed about pumps — thankfully.

One of our first stops was our pharmacy, where we were told that insulin pumps are not handled by drugstores. A few days later, however, our pharmacist called and said she had the business card of a pump distributor based in New Brunswick that had been passed to her by a satisfied pump user. We called Melany Hellstern of Disetronic Medical Systems, Inc. She sent us a kit filled with information, which we read over. Now we were really excited.

In the meantime, Dr. Dornan had recommended a pump from another manufacturer, so we called and obtained an information kit from that company, too, which we also studied.

Melany followed up and suggested that we should have a hands-on demonstration of insulin pumps so that we really knew what was involved. As it happened we were going to be passing through Fredericton, where she was based at the time, so she invited us for a demonstration.

It is important to acknowledge where Jack was in his diabetic journey at that point in time. He had lost a lot of vision. In fact his driving privileges had been reduced to local driving in Prince Edward Island, daytime only. He was having trouble reading and seeing in general. At times he had trouble concentrating and taking things in because of how he felt.

She spent three hours with us. She gave us not only information about the pump but also tremendous input about carbohydrate counting and living with diabetes in general. She was one of several miracles in our lives over those few weeks.

One of the most important things that Melany did was to sit Jack down at a table, hand him a pump, and get him actually doing all of the things he would have to become comfortable with doing. Remember, he had limited vision. He had to feel comfortable working with the pump. So did I, because we felt that he could be blind in a very short time. I had to be able to take over his insulin whether he was on the needle or the pump.

We both found the Disetronic pump quite easy to operate and not intimidating. Melany gave us the other pump that had been recommended to us and did a complete demonstration on it. She then left the room and asked us to go through the steps needed to operate both pumps on our own. We did. She gave us an opportunity to make up our minds, to work things through, from replacing batteries to loading insulin in the pump, to go through the procedure of changing the tubing and learning all of the mechanics of the pump, as well as to figure out how to enter the various settings, what the alarm codes mean, and so on.

We already had a basic knowledge because we had studied the material the pump companies sent, but this opportunity to sit down and try the different pumps, on our own and with no pressure, no one looking over our shoulder, was invaluable to us.

We made the decision to go with the Disetronic pump mainly based on Jack's vision problems. Here are some of the factors that made up our minds:

- The other pump had three batteries (the ones shaped like a dime), which had to be stacked in the right order and then placed in the pump. The marks indicating order were hard for Jack to see, and it was a fiddly procedure. The pump we chose has batteries that come in a drop-in little holder thingy so that we don't have to worry about the order or the fiddly stuff. Batteries are expensive, so this was an important point for us. The difficulties with the other model may have been rectified since we got our pump.

- The insulin in the other pump had to be drawn from a vial with a syringe, then injected into another vial that fit the pump. As part of the procedure care had to be taken that no air bubbles got into the lines that take the insulin from the pump to the body. It was a similar process to tapping the syringe to ensure that no air is injected into the body when using the needle, except now you were dealing with an even harder to see narrow plastic tube. The pump we chose takes a cartridge of short-acting insulin that is simply placed into the machine. Again, for Jack it was less fiddly, faster, and easier to do.

- He found the controls on the pump we chose easier to use because the buttons are raised.

- And finally — a huge factor for us — when we purchased our pump from Disetronic we received two pumps — one to use and a backup. The pumps have to go in for checkups, just like cars, and like all mechanical things there is a chance of accident or breakdown. Without a backup, Jack would have to go back to injecting with a needle while his pump was away for repair. We did not like that idea.

Once the decision was made we had to get a prescription from a diabetes specialist in one of a few hospitals accredited in Canada by our insurance company. Saint John Regional Hospital is one of them. And that doctor had to fill in a form and provide his credentials for the insurer. That information was sent off, and then we had to wait for approval before ordering our pump.

Once we had written approval from our insurance company, the pump provider would ship the pump and bill the insurer for their portion. We just had to pay our 20 percent. Even so, that 20 percent of the pump and a few months' supplies came to more than $2,000.

There were dozens of phone calls, letters, and appointments involved in this process that took several weeks.

As all of this was going on, we were in training for Jack's move to pumping and experienced something that truly led us to understand how important knowledge and management are.

Interpreting the disease and understanding how it affects you or those in your care is an important part of living with diabetes. This is not a disease that can be defined symptom by symptom in a textbook. It affects different people in different ways. Many factors come into play: age, stage of life, maturity, what people do for a living, how far it has progressed, environment, etc. How one individual reacts to a certain situation can be vastly different from another. The best way to cope is by mapping and acknowledging which factors affect you and in what way. Sometimes that is difficult to do, especially when dealing with young people.

BEYOND THE OBVIOUS

TA of Prince Edward Island has two sons with Type 1 diabetes. One of them has to take insulin daily; the other isn't on insulin yet because his diabetes is not yet fully developed. The boys were diagnosed in 2000 and 2004 respectively.

"Initially before diagnosis of our oldest son we thought he had leukemia and so we were actually thankful that it was diabetes. Then of course you always worry if they don't take their Dexasol with them, will they go low, will they go blind, etc."

The family finds frustration and challenges to be a part of living with youngsters with diabetes. "The most frustrating was when the diabetic centre told our son he could eat anything he liked in moderation," says TA. "Sounds okay, but I'd ask them not to tell him that, since moderation and our son don't get along. We had his diabetes regulated since he only ate what he was given, no junk food, etc. Now we find candy bar wrappers, chip bags, etc., hidden in his room." The most challenging? "The hardest is getting him to eat at regular times and consistent recording of his blood sugars."

"We realize we only have a few years to get him eating right before he is out on his own," TA says, and so they are working to instill good habits and responsibility in their boys. Their advice to others in a similar situation with children is, "Be firm in demanding they be responsible and take charge of their diabetic care. For example to take Dexasol or other sugar substitutes with them at all times. Eat regular and on time to help regulate their insulin/blood sugar levels. We do our children no favours by letting them do what they want — we only risk their future."

They didn't stop with the obvious. "The other things we did: removed the TV from our house, bought a health centre membership, and encourage fitness at every turn. We also hope to sign our son up for the islet replacement in Edmonton when he turns eighteen."

BE PROACTIVE

Making a few changes that make you feel better is relatively easy. The trick is to go beyond so that you're building your knowledge and finding things that work for you. There is a wealth of information available from sources we have discussed before. It is my belief that you have to take charge and go beyond the standard information.

With the objective of slowing the disease progression down, explore every piece of information. Discuss it with your doctor. I have long been aware of vitamins, foods, and such that are said to have specific benefits. For example, we read about a new mix of vitamins that had been developed to help slow down eye disease. I checked with both our family doctor and my eye specialist. The eye specialist highly recommended them for both Jack and I. Our family physician checked to ensure there was no conflict with the extensive drugs Jack is taking. With their approval we added Vitalux to our regime. (There are several other brand name products being developed to help combat eye disease.)

A year later there is much more recognition of the benefits of this treatment for eye disease. We believe that Jack has seen some benefit from them. How I wish we had known about them years ago! So, yes, I pay attention to things I read or hear. I research and consider them. It is our firm belief that this is one way of taking control and responsibility. At least we are not passively doing nothing but waiting for the next diabetic complication.

Sometimes I feel like a true nag and hesitate to suggest Jack do something. But truth is I'm the reader/researcher in the family. For instance one day I read that there is a link between dental care and good health, especially in diabetics. He's one of those people who are blessed with teeth that never, ever get cavities or even look like they need a brush. So for me to start nagging that he had to brush three times a day freaked him out. But I did it. If I can gain him one hour of better health by nagging, then nag I will.

At the time of writing there are a number of things that bear thinking about, such as:

Dental

There is research being done that suggests that good dental health, taking care of teeth and gums, might prevent heart disease, diabetes, and more. It has to do with preventing infections and that sort of thing. So, since we are all supposed to brush and floss anyway, and since it makes sense, why not just practise good dental hygiene? Brush and floss and schedule regular checkups with your dentist. Ban plaque! It's an easy thing to do.

Blueberries

We've been hearing for quite a while now that blueberries are good for us. Research indicates they may have anti-diabetic properties. There is a school of thought that says our move away from natural foods like blueberries is part of the reason for the rise in diseases like diabetes. When Jack was recently hospitalized for surgery his post-operation guidelines recommended drinking blueberry or cranberry juice. When I was researching ways to help Jack's eyes I discovered that the bilberry, a European cousin to our blueberry, had been used for years over the pond. In fact bilberry was given to fighter pilots in the Second World War to improve their night vision. Now my feeling is that there has to be something to all of this. So, a scoop of blueberries with your morning cereal or a blueberry dessert: as long as you count them in your diet, why not!

Another place where knowledge works is in making your diet work for you. Eating is a vital part of our lives, so why not make it as palatable as possible? The key to maintaining a good healthy diet is to understand what goes past your lips.

Sugar substitutes

If you have a true penchant for sweets, diabetes can be very difficult. We have a proliferation of supposedly sugar-free products out there — many of which simply disguise the sugar. New labelling regulations will help with that one. There are sugar substitutes that give foods a sweet taste without affecting your blood sugar. They can be sprinkled on, stirred in, and even used in cooking. They are also used in products such as soft drinks, yogurts, etc. To learn about the various sugar substitutes, go to an education training session led by a diabetes educator.

But, do remember, the trouble with these products is that they perpetuate your taste, your desire, for sweet foods. Why not let yourself discover the real flavours of foods? Once you get past the need for that sugar taste you might be surprised at the delights that await you.

Sugar smarts

Sugars do not have to be looked at as poison that must be eliminated from your life. For starters they are naturally part of many fruits, vegetables, and such that are necessary sources of energy. If you follow a healthy, well-balanced meal plan with a variety of foods you can include sugars in your diet as part of your total carbohydrate intake. It is important that they be used in moderation and be counted into your carbohydrate intake — not just added on as extras.

Carb smarts

Smart folks learn about carbohydrates. One of three major sources of energy used by our bodies (along with fat and protein), carbohydrates come in different forms, which include starch, sugars, and fibre. Confused? The Canadian Diabetes Association has loads of information about sugars. It says:

- Starch is found in cereals, bread, pasta, and vegetables like corn, potatoes, and legumes.
- Sugars are found naturally in fruits, vegetables, and milk.
- Sugar is found naturally in refined sugars such as the white stuff you put on the table, brown sugar, or icing sugar.
- Fibre adds bulk through foods like whole grain products, fruits, and vegetables.
- All carbohydrates end up as glucose, or sugar, in the blood to be used as a source of energy. The body doesn't know the difference between natural or added sugars. It doesn't have the capability of checking incoming sugar and deciding which is good and which is bad. It's up to you — the thinking you — to determine the source of your energy and how it affects your health.

Fibre and carbs

When you go to educational sessions today dieticians will talk to you about counting carbs and subtracting fibre to maintain good control. I'm not going to write about that because Jack doesn't do the subtracting fibre thing. Although it is now being taught, we were told that he is doing so well with the counting methods he has developed that he should carry on as he is doing. He has a system for dealing with things that are high fibre, like pasta and rice — things that tend to break down slowly. He tests his blood an extra time, one to two hours after eating, and if necessary he takes more insulin.

It comes down to looking at what you are eating and really thinking about it. Is there a lot of fibre? Is it quick energy that will drive sugars up fast but won't last? Think about what you eat. Aim for balance. If you just don't know what is in food, then find out. These days between label requirements and excellent resource material the answers are there.

Although there is a proliferation of "stuff" about counting carbs available today, we recommend the paperback *The Corinne T. Netzer Carbohydrate Counter* (ISBN 0-440-23682-7) or one of the companion books published by Dell Publishing in the United States. This author also published *The Complete Book of Food Counts* and several others. Take a few minutes to check the inside pages to see which suits your needs and is easy for you to read and understand.

It sounds complicated, but after a while you get to know what works for you and what doesn't. That is what it all comes down to — learning how you can best maintain control.

"Carb counting is the best way, with fibre being subtracted," said our diabetes educator, "but if it's going to confuse the patient then they have to come up with what works for them."

Some, especially the elderly, have trouble if it gets too complicated, so aim for a simple system and slowly add things to fine-tune it.

EATING OUT AND EATING IN

I never thought I would say it, but fast food restaurants are often your best bet if you need to stay in control. The reason is simple. Most have nutrition charts that tell you the carbs, fat, protein, etc., in every standard menu item. It may not be the healthiest food, but at least you know what you are dealing with, and by consulting the chart you can make the best choices.

In finer dining restaurants the portions are not usually big enough to be a huge problem, but if you are concerned about the quantity of food turn to the appetizer menu. It's a trick food writers use. We do it to allow ourselves to sample different dishes without overindulging and breaking the bank. Many appetizers are mini portions of main dishes and much less expensive.

Restaurant eating is hard, but what is harder is being invited to eat at someone's home. At restaurants a person can look at the menu and choose something that is close to what they should have. When invited to someone's home for a sit-down meal there is no control over timing or ingredients.

People brush off the importance of the timing. We have actually had to leave dinner parties and go to restaurants because the meal that had been promised for six o'clock was not on the table by eight. That kind of scenario is upsetting for all — the hostess, who either feels guilty or thinks you are out to ruin her party; the diabetic, who is put in a position of calling attention to his disease and can become ill in the process; others present, who are often embarrassed; and those like me — forced into the position of being the witch, the fierce mother protector, the fanatical wife.

By now I'm sure readers are tired of my preaching the importance of taking responsibility, of using knowledge to help maintain control and fight for quality of life. Sorry about that. The reality is that it is so important, not just to the diabetic, but also to everyone who is affected by what goes on in the diabetic's life. I had originally planned to place the following personal account in chapter three, where we discussed the impact on others. But then I realized that this father's denial, his refusal to do the things we've talked about, is a prime example of what not to do — and a real inspiration for diabetics to get with the program. Think about whether you want your actions — or inaction — to put your family through this kind of lifelong experience.

DENIAL CAUSES CONSTANT WORRY

AC of Ontario faces the problems that many people living with a diabetic in denial have to cope with. Her father, a Type 1 diabetic for more than forty years, has a daily routine of insulin and diet regulation (low-sodium and low-sugar).

Where her father differs from many other diabetics is in the support group he has around him. He is almost a casebook study in his approach to his health and his failure to acknowledge how his actions affect his family and to take steps to alleviate their concerns. AC shares her story.

"My father's diabetes has been very stressful for my immediate family — I have three siblings — especially my mother who has spent her entire marriage looking after my dad, helping to monitor his diet, preparing his food, ensuring he is taking his medication, and desperately trying to help him become more active about his own health.

"The situation has become increasingly worse over the years, especially now that my dad is getting older (he will be turning sixty this year). In the last year he has suffered a massive heart attack, had eye surgery on one eye and awaits surgery on the other, increased circulation problems affecting his lower limbs, and several insulin shock episodes.

"This has been scary for us because we do not live in the same cities and we are in constant fear that something terrible will happen. The most difficult part of this lifelong process is convincing my father to learn to take care of himself. In a large part I believe he is still in a long stage of denial and thus often forgets to eat at scheduled times and administer insulin at scheduled times. This has been frustrating to no end."

Her father is probably a caring individual who would never do anything to harm or upset his family, yet his actions, or perhaps I should say his inaction, are doing just that.

"Increasingly I have become more scared, especially because my father is aging. Just last week we went to the emergency because he had lost track of time and went into insulin shock, collapsing on the floor. This is terrifying because if this were to happen while he was alone somewhere, he could very well possibly die.

"The most frustrating thing is his unwillingness to really understand and regulate his disease. He has a loving wife and four loving children that take care of him, and he neglects to understand how serious his condition is and, at the same time, how manageable it is.

I find that he is in part in denial and in part reliant on others to ensure his well-being. I love my father, but sometimes I really feel that he has caused a lot of suffering within the family because of his lack of common sense and accountability for his diabetes.

"The most challenging part is not being in the same city. I live in Toronto and my parents live in Kingston. It would be nice to be closer so that I could help him monitor and regulate his disease."

One stress family members have that comes with the territory is a feeling of responsibility for keeping "their" diabetic healthy. AC concurred. "Absolutely! With this disease comes responsibility and guilt. I hate to be an overbearing person or bossy but often I feel as though I am parenting my own father."

Does that lead to an overwhelming concern about timing, meals, or overall health?

"Oh yes. In every phone conversation or in-person visit, my first question will be regarding his diabetes — how is he feeling overall, did he eat, when did he eat, what is his blood sugar level currently, etc. My father's health is visibly deteriorating, so myself and everyone else in the family is constantly worrying."

So what does AC do to help herself and her family cope with her father's illness? For starters, she tries to learn as much as she can by reading a lot on the subject. Whenever possible she or one of her siblings accompanies him to appointments.

"We talk a lot as a family, minus my dad, about his situation, how to improve things, how to help him. It really helps to have the support of my family in discussing these things as I find often that people without a diabetic loved one don't understand the severity of this disease."

This diabetic gets lots of support and special encouragement in an attempt to get him to take charge of his diabetes.

"We gently coax him to read more about his disease, try to make him understand how much it stresses and hurts our family that he neglects his disease. I will remind him often to test his blood sugar levels, ensure he is making his appointments. And on special occasions, when I am home, I will give my dad a nice leg and foot rub to help his circulation and tell him how much I love him."

AC offers advice for others who have a diabetic in their family:

- Read as much as you can on diabetes and provide reading materials for your diabetic to read.
- Accompany your diabetic to doctor's appointments or counselling sessions if you can.
- Seek help from others in your situation. Talking to others who live what you live really helps.
- Make sure you take time for yourself.

If AC's father had been born a generation earlier there is little doubt that he would not have survived to age sixty as a Type 1 diabetic. He is proof positive of the value of a support team. His family and medical professionals must be credited.

There is no doubt in my mind that knowledge is power. In fact I had grand plans of passing along knowledge of food and things like fibre and starches and proper diet. The more I read the more I realized I don't know. I also realized that so much of this diabetes thing is figuring out what works for each individual.

Not everyone has the same response to every food, so it's important to figure out your own plan, your own targets. A lot of that comes down to trial and error. If you eat potatoes and test your blood an hour and a half later and it's in a good range, then you can tolerate potatoes. If peas or corn puts your sugars up, then you know you can't tolerate them easily.

There is much more to understand and interpret than eating. At an annual meeting of the Prince Edward Island chapter of the Canadian Diabetes Association, Dr. Gary Costain was the guest speaker. While I said I was not going to get input from medical professionals for this book, this was a public meeting and his message to a general audience. Folks like us.

He said he was going to take the opportunity to talk to the audience the way he would like to be able to talk to every one of his patients if only he had the time. Obviously what I have cited below is excerpted from a long speech. It is food for thought and, I think, demonstrates how important it is to work with professionals in managing your diabetes. You should also note that I did not include what was said about specific drugs because that type of information has to be between you and your professional team.

THE DOCTOR'S VIEW

"A lot of people think all we are trying to do is prevent blindness and kidney failure. But what causes the most suffering and death and trauma are vascular complications. We need to stop heart attacks and strokes.

"You can't just concentrate on blood sugars. It's a full meal deal. Unfortunately people are going to be on a lot of pills and that can be expensive. You may be surprised at the list." However, he says, "If a patient is worth treating, and worth treating well, they will end up on a lot of pills and medications."

"Count up risk factors present. If we develop an aggressive approach we can do more."

He referred to treatment of diabetes as a "multi-factor intervention," which includes diet, exercise, stopping smoking, regulating glucose, monitoring things like blood pressure and cholesterol, as well as taking medications.

"I have a checklist when I see patients which includes: diet and exercise, smoking cessation, ASA (81 mg daily), A1C sugar control, blood sugars, ACE inhibitors, lipids and statins to lower cholesterol.

"The number one priority — stop smoking." Smoking dramatically increases risk for diabetics and is, he says, something that we can do something about. "Stopping makes a big difference." He pointed out that the money saved can be applied to the ACE inhibitors and statins you may need.

"The number two priority — get moving. We do not do enough health counselling in our society to get people moving. We need to help people exercise in keeping with their ability. Even if they don't lose weight, all exercise will decrease risk."

Activity has no cost, but, says Dr. Costain, give up a medium coffee and a donut and you will save ten dollars a week that can go towards buying a treadmill. The purchase of a treadmill is, he says, "the one piece of advice people come back and thank me for. Everyone in the house can use it — just make sure they do."

"Take a multivitamin — it may reduce infections in diabetics. There is no harm to taking one or two multivitamins a day and it's not expensive. Some tend to make people nauseated — try another one. Vitamin D is necessary, and in this part of the world in all but July and August you should be supplementing.

"Keep your blood pressure in control; it is as important as lowering sugars. Get to always reading 130 (if attainable, 120) over 80. If you can't do that with diet and exercise, then you need medication. Taking steps to lower blood pressure has more effect than lowering sugars. In this part of the world probably 25 percent of heart attacks are related to insulin resistance."

As for those blood sugars: "Getting A1C from 12 to 11 percent can reduce risk by 18 percent. People don't like to take multiple medications. We are working to break that barrier and get people on medications they need. It's an adding in sort of thing."

His guideline for exercise: "Just do it. Everyone has enough time for exercise."

He suggests the equivalent of walking for at least twenty minutes a day, five days a week, or, if healthy enough, "a run is probably better in the long term." He also recommends weightlifting because the benefits are longer term: it increases metabolism for two or three days, whereas walking increases metabolism only while you are doing it. Be realistic, he says. "That is how we were designed: to forage for food, to walk a lot, to run away from predators, to lift and carry."

And, we are stuck with what we are. "It's too late to get yourself adopted out. You're stuck with your genes."

Remember, treatment depends on the condition of the individual, his or her age, and many other factors. Each individual is unique and must work out a personal plan, including lifestyle changes, with his or her physician.

HEMOGLOBIN A1C

When talking diabetes and management plans and control the term A1C is often dropped into the conversation. So what is it? The hemoglobin A1C is a simple lab test that uses a small sample of blood to show how well you have controlled your blood glucose levels over the past three months by "calculating" your average daily blood glucose reading.

Doctors use the hemoglobin A1C blood test, also called GHb and glycated hemoglobin, to determine long-term control of blood glucose levels.

Checking blood glucose levels at home with your own monitor is the first way to know if your blood glucose readings are in the target range and gives you short-term control.

A1C tests are usually done two to three times a year. If they are not suggested, ask for them and then discuss the results with your doctor. Don't assume that a good A1C means you have no problems. If there are things you feel aren't right, tell your doctor.

If your A1C is high your doctor may ask you to monitor and record your blood glucose levels more frequently each day in an effort to identify when they are up. Then you both can work for better control.

Don't think you can get away with not finger pricking because you have had an A1C. Checking with your own tester reveals how food, exercise, and diabetes medicines affect your blood sugar, which the A1C test cannot show. Each test provides very different sets of information, and both are needed to help control your diabetes and thus help you lower your risk of complications.

Can't be bothered to make changes? Think about this one. "Preventable diet and inactivity related diseases (such as diabetes) lead to an estimated 20-47,000 premature deaths every year in Canada." (*Homemakers Magazine*, May 2004 issue.)

There is so much information out there about things one should and should not do that it gets confusing. The reality is that the media love to sensationalize. They are interested in "news" — a fast hit — a headline. So, if you hear something that seems to be interesting or that might be useful to you, investigate further and discuss it with your doctor.

Having said that, there are many things reported that are useful reminders. For instance, on September 11, 2004, I read a report in the *Moncton Times Transcript* stating that women who drink more than one sweetened soft drink a day are slightly more likely to develop diabetes than women who drink less than one a month, a finding that came from a study reported in the *Journal of the American Medical Association* that saw 51,603 female nurses analyzed.

The article said that the Harvard University researchers who did the study reported that since obesity is strongly linked to Type 2 diabetes, the extra calories from the soda would account for at least some of the increased risk. But they said there also appears to be a link to the way the body handles sugars in soft drinks.

So what can the diabetic take from this news report? It's a wake-up call. A red flag. A "proceed with caution." That's what. Ever get tempted to have a real cola? Reach for the no-sugar kind instead. You don't want to compromise your weight or take the chance with "the way the body handles sugars in soft drinks."

GETTING YOUR RECORD STRAIGHT

Taking action is one of the most important things that you can do when it comes to living with diabetes. The positive vibes that you get are doing something for your own good, rather than passively sitting back and waiting for the worst to happen.

One of the positive things you can do is create your own medical history. Writing or recording your medical history and current information is something most of us neglect, but having it written down can save you time at critical moments. It's one of those jobs good to have done.

Recently Jack was admitted to the hospital for surgery. During his pre-op interview and tests the nurse wrote down details of things that happened forty years ago. She reminded us of things we had long forgotten. I got a copy of what she wrote out. Later I got it onto the computer, on a disk, and put a printed version in a file. So, why do we need to do this?

Much of the information physicians gather about you is used to make decisions about your care. The only source they have for that information is you. The last thing you want to do when you are sick is try to remember all this stuff. You'll probably forget something. Illness or an emergency strain your memory.

Include any conditions you might have: operations, past illnesses, allergies, hospitalizations, even immunizations if you can. Also include a listing of all the medications, including over-the-counter ones, that you take. Don't forget the vitamins and herbal preparations. These last two are important because they can interact with some drugs, and some of their natural results can do things like thin blood. You should also jot down significant illnesses of close relatives.

This kind of detailing might sound unnecessary, but remember that your own records, what you tell your doctors, are the tools they use to make their diagnosis. Having the proper information at hand will help everyone get the best results possible.

VISITS TO YOUR DOCTOR

These days, when doctors are stretched to the limit by huge patient lists, we have to make the best use possible of the time we spend with them. It is all too easy to forget questions or reasons for being there. There are several things you can do to best utilize the time you have with your physician. Your most important tools here are a pen and paper:

- Write down the reasons for your visit: a prescription refill, a specific pain, symptoms you need checked.
- Write down all of your questions.
- Write down all of your concerns, no matter how trivial they may seem.
- Keep a list going by your place at the table, and just before you go to the doctor's rewrite it, listing the most important reason for your visit — your biggest concerns or problems — at the top. Holding back serious issues until the end of your appointment means they can get less time and attention than they deserve!

- Check all of your medications to see if you need refills.
- Take a friend or family member in to see the doctor with you. They can do several things for you: listen and take notes, ask questions that you forget or are embarrassed to bring up, and act as an advocate for you.

THINGS ARE CHANGING? BE WARY

If your physician prescribes changes in how you manage your diabetes, be sure to take extra care during the transition period. Mistakes are more easily made when you change from your normal routine or at turning points in treatment. You must understand the changes: how you are to make them, why you are making them, what these changes will do, both to your health and how you feel, and what you should expect to happen.

If your doctor prescribes a prescription change, take your supply of the old medications to the pharmacy and ask your pharmacist to dispose of what you should not be taking. Don't keep them around. Also be sure to update your records. Ask your pharmacist for an updated printout of what you are taking for your files and medical information. Change appropriate things, like MedicAlert information.

Pay close attention to the directions that come with new prescriptions and follow them carefully. Remember, you have to unlearn what went before and learn a new routine. It can take a few days.

Finally, pay attention to your medications, treatments, and necessary details:

- Know what they look like and what they do.
- Know how many pills you take at what times.
- Know how much insulin you are supposed to take.
- Know the names of your doctors.
- Know key medical terms for the conditions you have.

I know. By now your eyes are rolling back in your head or you are shaking that head back and forth in disbelief. How can one individual be expected to do all of this stuff — to know it all, to practise all of these things?

> Follow your instincts. If you think or feel that something is not right, it probably isn't. Talk to members of your support team and push till you get answers.

Just remember the rule: one step at a time. You will amaze yourself at how quickly you can do these things, and do them well, if you just set your mind to it.

THE WORD-OF-MOUTH NETWORK

One of the best ways to gain knowledge and put aside collywobbles is by talking to others. It is important to remember that you are not alone. There is a network out there; you just have to take a few initial steps to become part of it.

Today the phone rang in our house. It was a fellow from Hamilton, Ontario, who had heard about Jack's experiences with the insulin pump and called for information. "It's great. I play golf now and everything," Jack began before going into the details of how the pump works, how the individual works with the pump, and so on. "Got started on it, got following the new routine, and I've been sailing ever since." Months earlier Jack had been the one phoning to ask questions from someone else.

In the doctor's office Jack often ends up chatting to people — these days about the pump. They recognize him from the picture of him that appeared in an article the local newspaper did about Jack and his pump. This day several other diabetics were in the waiting room of the eye specialist. Because of the long wait, one gal had to go to a nearby store and buy something to eat. Her blood sugars were low. That triggered conversation about the benefits of the pump, an important one being the flexibility that it gives.

Another great way to learn and meet people is by attending courses put on by dieticians in grocery stores or community centres. I attended three hour-long sessions spread over three weeks called

Healthy Eating for Diabetes Management. It cost ten dollars and lunch was included in the last session. These sessions focused on things like understanding sweeteners, reading labels, and, on the final day, cooking tips, a demo, recipes, and lunch.

I have to stress that you must take the information given at store-endorsed sessions as guidelines only, not gospel truth. Keep in mind that the dieticians work for the store and are there to promote its products. At one session I noticed errors in what the dietician said about counting the carbs in pasta. But most upsetting to me was a statement that "most of you here are just on pills so you don't have to worry about being too accurate."

That scared me. I feel that you have to be very careful at this stage to build good habits, not be encouraged to be slack in management. It was a personal thing from my point of view.

But also keep in mind why you should attend such sessions. Learning about various sweeteners and how to read labels and meeting other diabetics was a very positive way to spend a few hours of my time. The dietician also addressed fibre and helped to open people's eyes about the many products out there that claim to be low-carb but are overpriced and loaded with fat.

One young woman was there because she wanted to know more about diabetes for her diabetic father. She also felt that she should learn as much about diabetes as she could since it was in the family. She arranged for an early lunch hour so that she and her father could attend together. Smart gal. Her dad, who had been diagnosed five years previously, said he felt a need to keep fresh every year because things change. Smart guy.

KEEP IT FRESH AND FRIENDLY

I'm not going to dwell on diets. You get enough of that. There is loads of information out there about what to eat, when to eat, and how to cook it. Counting carbs and reducing fat are part of your life.

The one comment I will make is to urge you to beware of becoming bored or tired of your special eating program. If you restrict your eating to the point where boredom sets in you may well find yourself in trouble. Forbidden goodies will tempt you, and it's easy to give in just one time. That one time is okay if you can limit it to an occasional treat, but all too often when one sneak is okay, when you don't suffer ill affects from it, you start to get lax. A slip here, a slip there, then one day you realize you are in trouble. Blood sugars are not where they should be. You have lost your dietary edge.

One of the keys to fight that boredom is to embrace your eating program by learning to prepare and eat a wide variety of foods, paying attention to portion sizes so that they become the norm. Try new things. With a little effort you can enjoy a lifetime of healthy eating that is enjoyable and satisfying.

Work out a listing of snacks and treats that you can enjoy so that you are prepared when a craving hits.

At first, reading labels, measuring or weighing food, and learning new ways to cook might seem too much of a challenge, too time consuming. But you soon get used to it. These are the tools. One diabetic I know made up a book where she kept carb counts of their favourite foods. A smart move.

We have done a similar thing, but we have another tool that has been a wonderful help to us. When we were researching the possibility of Jack obtaining an insulin pump the representative from the pump company recommended a book that she found invaluable in the care of her young son, a pump user: *The Corinne T. Netzer Carbohydrate Counter*.

We carry that book around with us. To give you an idea of how we use it, picture a Chinese buffet. A couple of times a month we head on over to the Magic Wok. We are probably the only customers they have who come in with a pen, paper, and carb-counting book, but that is what we do.

Jack will get his food and then make a note of what he has on the paper. I usually look up the carbs for anything he doesn't know as he's going. He has things like broccoli, steamed mussels, and egg rolls down pat, but anything new we look up.

Jack's routine on the insulin pump is to test before eating, then he eats his meal, counting carbs, and at the end of the meal he takes a shot of insulin to compensate for what he ate. In a case like this where we eat out and where we are guessing at some of the carbs, he tests again in two hours and makes any insulin adjustment necessary. If his sugars are up at all he will take another bolus of insulin.

By writing down what he has to eat each time he goes up to the buffet he is very aware of what he is eating and how much. The running total of carbs is a real indicator that, hey, I've had enough.

In the old days a buffet meant half a dozen trips to fill his plate. That was twenty-five years ago. Today he still makes three or four trips, but he will come back each time with just a few items on his plate. Things that he loves like olives and chicken wings will be savoured and enjoyed to the fullest. Today quality, not quantity, rules. Best of all, Jack can go to the buffet with a group of people and truly enjoy both the company and the eating experience.

He no longer walks away feeling like he has a rock in his gut. He's satisfied, but he doesn't overeat. Since going on the insulin pump the only reaction he has had to a Chinese buffet is going a bit low — which he quickly counteracts — because he counted a couple of things as having more carbs than they did. We now have those figured out and he's so accurate that he gets a bit smug about it.

CHAPTER 7

Taking Charge by Becoming Your Own Advocate

When Jack took an early retirement at age sixty, we honestly didn't think he was going to have much life left to live. We pinned our hopes for better days on his not having to work at a job that by its very nature made it difficult for him to maintain control of his diabetes, and on taking charge of as much of our life as possible. We were determined to find out as much as we could about treatments, ways to handle the disease, even how we should best live our day-to-day life.

By taking action, Jack turned his life in a better direction. This story might seem a bit long and convoluted, but bear with me. It's important because our pursuit of better control set things in motion that would have a dramatic effect on our quality of life. We didn't do anything difficult or have any special education. What we had was a will. Determination.

What I find scary is that we are not particularly good at taking on the establishment or aggressive about fighting for our rights. I envy those who are. And I'm frightened for those who are worse at it than we are.

How I wish that we had educated ourselves and become more involved with fighting this disease earlier. We probably could have slowed things down or even prevented some things. I will always wonder if we could have prevented Jack's rapid vision change if we had become proactive sooner.

When we finally did take action we not only experienced better health for Jack, but mentally we both felt so much better. There is nothing worse than feeling that you have no control over what is happening to you. There is a saying that the fear of the unknown is the greatest fear there is. When you don't know what you can do to help yourself, it seems like your life is spinning away, out of your control.

To tell our story, I feel the need to set the scene, as they say, so that you, the reader, can see how small steps taken towards a goal do eventually get you to a destination.

We had begun planning for Jack's retirement several years previously, putting as much money as we could into RSPs, moving into an easy-to-maintain home, and doing everything we could to maintain his health. We had looked at alternate medicine and had begun exploring the possibility of his getting an insulin pump.

At this point Jack was having trouble controlling his blood sugars and was often exhausted — to the point where I would have to help him up the stairs — and suffering with kidney problems, frequent angina, and more.

A vacation seemed a good way to start retirement, and for him to de-stress from work. We hadn't been able to take a holiday for years. His vacation time had always been used for sick days or for family emergencies. So, we bravely set of for British Columbia.

Jack was not really well, but we worked hard to keep him in control and well rested. He was tired when we boarded the plane home but generally pleased with our vacation. Retirement was agreeing with him.

Unfortunately taking to the air did not. Jack's diabetic body just didn't seem able to handle the lack of oxygen or the four-hour time difference. By the time we got home I was seriously worried. Jack reacted badly to the flight and complicated his recovery by succumbing to the flu. He ended up down for three weeks. The symptoms were familiar. Flu combined with total exhaustion. He would wake up tired, so tired that it took every ounce of his effort to get out of bed and to the bathroom. He would seem to improve a little once he was up, but not much. I watched the clock and roused him to check his sugars and eat.

He had experienced these symptoms before, but this time we had a major concern. Two weeks after getting home he had an appointment with the eye specialist. He was really too ill to go out, but at the same time he didn't want to miss his appointment because it would take months to get another.

Jack had had lens replacements and laser treatments for bleeds in his eyes. His vision had been good in British Columbia. He drove most of the time while I navigated, the same as we have always done. But now, when he was so ill, his eyes were like the rest of his body — not at their best.

After a brief exam, the eye specialist picked up his tape recorder and dictated a letter to the Department of Motor Vehicles withdrawing Jack's driving privileges. Jack tried to explain that he was ill. He asked for another appointment, but nothing would budge the eye specialist. Not once in that appointment did he ask about Jack's diabetes, his insulin routine, or anything else relating to the fact that he was ill.

This is an example of a situation where diabetics have to become their own advocates. Our medical system does not allow time for physicians to consult about patients or to take the team approach that would be ideal for those with multiple conditions where diabetes is a common denominator.

You need to fight your own battles. You need to be the central hub, the one who does know that common denominator. In this case, we knew that the condition he was in was not normal. We knew his eyes had deteriorated, but not to that degree. Something just didn't feel right about the diagnosis.

At about the same time, one of our efforts started to gel into action. Jack had asked our doctor for a referral to explore the possibility of his getting an insulin pump. A phone call came making an appointment for him to go to Saint John, New Brunswick, to be evaluated for the pump.

Days later a letter arrived from Motor Vehicles restricting Jack to driving in the daytime, locally (in our case that meant in Prince

Edward Island) only, and requesting that he present himself for evaluation to see if he could retain even those driving privileges. We went to their office, explained our situation, and requested that the evaluation be delayed until after he had been evaluated in Saint John. The delay was approved and Jack agreed to in-province, daytime driving only in the meantime.

The tale of Jack's insulin pump experience appears in the next chapter, but exciting things started happening even before his startup. After his evaluation in Saint John and approval for pump therapy, Jack and I were scheduled for educational sessions on carbohydrate counting — a mandatory part of pump therapy.

When we returned home to Prince Edward Island we once again went to Motor Vehicles and explained about the education sessions, which would be followed by his going on the pump. Once again they agreed to wait to test for his driver's licence. Jack agreed to

---

THE DAWN PHENOMENON

Have you ever experienced a situation where your blood sugars tested normal when you went to bed but had increased to read high by the time you got up, even though you had not eaten anything? If so, you have probably experienced the "dawn phenomenon," a rising blood sugar level that occurs approximately between 3:00 a.m. and the time of waking up.

The way I understand it, the liver is supposed to release just enough sugar to replace what is being used, and insulin works as the messenger to tell the liver how much is enough. But if there's not enough insulin (as in Type 1 diabetes), or if there's enough insulin but it cannot communicate its messages to the liver (as in Type 2 diabetes), the liver starts to release sugar much too fast. As a result blood sugar levels rise, even if you haven't eaten a thing.

The danger is that this rise is not always good for the body. You should discuss your blood sugars with your doctor if you notice that they are high in the morning. Before you head off to the doc's office, do some intensive record-keeping for a few days. As well as your log of blood sugar readings, which should include both a before-bed and an on-waking test, record what you ate and when, when you took medications and what they were, and any physical activity. Changes to your routine or medications may well be in order.

continue to abide by the restrictions of driving only in the province during the day.

In late November we returned to Saint John for training on carbohydrate counting. They also evaluated his current insulin regime and made some changes to how he took his insulin. At that time Jack was injecting both long- and short-acting insulin — a total of six needles every day.

The doctor changed the time of his long-acting insulin from 6:00 p.m. to 10:00 p.m., explaining that he was taking the long-acting too early and thus suffering from the dawn phenomenon. It was the first time we had heard the term.

After a day of classes on carbohydrate counting we headed out, hoping to avoid the cost of another night in a hotel. We left Saint John for the five-hour trip home at about 4:00 p.m. The sun was shining and a light snow was just starting to fall. We were heading away from the city, so rush-hour traffic wasn't bad on the four-lane highway. Within a few miles the temperature dropped dramatically and we began one of the worst drives of my life.

The first inkling of trouble came with a slight slip of the back end of the car when we drove over a bridge. I dropped our speed and pulled in behind a snowplow that was putting salt on the road. All seemed to be okay, so after a couple of miles I pulled out to pass and got a fast lesson on the dangers of black ice. Two SUVs spun out of control ahead of us and a pickup braked too fast and did the same thing. I eased off the gas and tucked back in behind the snowplow. Obviously no one was hurt, so I just kept going. The road conditions were horrendous, but this stretch had nowhere to pull off.

I still take pride in the way I drove that day. We crept along, but I managed to keep our van on the road, unlike dozens of cars, trucks, tractor-trailers, and even more SUVs that hit the ditches. At the exit to Sussex, I eased onto the off-ramp and pulled into a parking lot. I was shaking and I think Jack was as well. I simply refused to go any further, saw a motel across the street, and gingerly drove over, sliding into a parking space with great relief.

After a few minutes spent composing ourselves we addressed the subject of supper. In those days Jack ate on time or he was in trouble. Since I couldn't face driving again, we had a choice of McDonald's or Kentucky Fried Chicken. We opted for chicken. Anyone who watches food in relation to diabetes will tell you that KFC tastes wonderful but makes it very hard to regulate blood sugar levels, presumably because of the high fat.

With the box of chicken sitting on the table between us, Jack said, "Well, I guess we'll try this new insulin routine and carb counting. We have nothing else to do but try to figure it out."

It had been explained to us that the instructions we had received to take his long-acting insulin at suppertime were wrong. He was to take the long-acting later in the evening to compensate for the dawn phenomenon that was causing so many of Jack's problems. He was also to count his carbs and take insulin calculated by what he ate, rather than a set amount before a meal. We did our best.

Out came the carb-counting book and instructions from the hospital. Jack checked this list and the book and counted the carbs as best he could. He injected his long-acting insulin at the later time and we snuggled in to enjoy a movie. It was so nice to be cozy and warm, safe in our comfy bed.

I woke up feeling refreshed, but not eager to crawl out of the covers. Then I heard something strange. Whistling. Jack was sitting up in bed, leaning against the headboard, whistling while he watched television. Weird. He was cheerful and alert. Weirder.

And he was watching television from across the room.

At breakfast in the lobby Jack was exuberant, keeping up a chattering observation of the ice-clearing and sanding activities outside. He bustled outside to scrape the ice from the car while I packed our bag. Soon we deemed the roads fit and were back on the four-lane highway heading to Moncton.

"There's a truck ahead," he said. Sure enough a way down the highway there was a truck.

"I see it, dear."

"The speed limit's 110."

"I know, dear."

"Moncton, eighty kilometres."

"Is that all."

"The lanes are merging, you need to get over."

"Yes, dear!"

He rambled on with his road observations till finally he turned to me in exasperation and said, "You don't get it, do you!"

Oh, I got it all right. I had been waiting for him to acknowledge it.

"I can see the traffic! I can read the road signs!"

I had been thanking God and Dr. Dornan and Linda Graham at Saint John Regional Hospital since the moment I heard him whistling. Since I saw him watching TV from further than eight feet away. Since I sat in a coffee shop in a hotel lobby and saw animation as he watched people outside the window. Since he warned me of an approaching truck, read a road sign, and checked the speed limit. Since I got the hint that my Jack, the old Jack that I love so well, was in there and starting to emerge again.

I swear we grinned all the way home.

Every day it seemed things got a little better. With this great beginning we couldn't wait for the next step.

Jack's eyes had improved so much that at his next appointment the eye specialist agreed to lift the restrictions on his licence. We waited while his staff prepared the information, then drove straight over to Motor Vehicles. Presented with his new readings they immediately reinstated full driving privileges, expressing delight that his treatments had been satisfactory.

Jack's vision is not perfect, but he has been given time — time to enjoy life, to get his health in better order, and to do everything possible to ensure that he maintains as much vision as he can for as long as he can. At the time of this writing he is still driving. He has to have his eyes checked regularly, but that is a small price to pay for the privilege of retaining his driver's licence.

Several weeks later, when we returned to the hospital for Jack's pump startup, we told Dr. Dornan of the wonderful change that had occurred. We thanked him and Linda Graham profusely for the miracle they had given us when they corrected how Jack was taking his long-acting insulin and started him counting carbs. We were especially grateful for the improvement in Jack's vision — and for the feeling of hope for the future.

Neither Jack nor I will ever forget Dr. Dornan's words when we expressed our gratitude.

"We've started working on the front of the eyes," he said, "now we'll get started on the back."

So, having reached the end of this tale, I'm sure many of you are asking where the education and advocacy come in.

Looking back we realized that we should have taken charge earlier. For example, he should not have kept his appointment with the eye specialist when he was so ill. But that is a hard call when you are being treated for something as valuable as your eyes and know you won't get another appointment for months.

We did the right thing in our dealings with Motor Vehicles. We did the right thing in educating ourselves about insulin pumps and jumping through all of the hoops put out by bureaucrats and insurance companies.

There are a few things that it is important for me to point out here. First and foremost, our relationship with the Department of Motor Vehicles, which issues driver's licences in our province, was excellent. The staff listened to what we had to say, worked with us by allowing Jack the time he needed to get on the pump, and, most importantly, we felt, the person we dealt with treated us with respect and dignity. I will always appreciate that.

The point is that even though they had sent the letter restricting driving privileges they were not the enemy and there was no personal grudge. We had a good relationship in part because of our own approach to them. We were polite. We had valid points to make. We did not act aggressively. At the same time we didn't lie down and passively let fate stomp on us without an effort on our own behalf.

It is terribly important to have the right approach when taking the role of advocate. It goes back to the team approach. By asking people to work with you, by acknowledging them as important players, you can count them in your team.

I also swelled with pride in my husband's approach to the whole thing. Don't get me wrong. He hated what was happening to him. He alternated between depression and anger. He was not a happy camper. But he was mature and responsible. He obeyed the rules as set down. Even though we went to Ontario in between our visits to Saint John Hospital, he did not drive out of province. Even locally, he pulled over a few times and asked me to drive because he did not feel he could see well enough to be behind the wheel.

It wasn't easy for Jack to relinquish control. He loves to drive. He loved touring on his motorcycle. When we were together he drove. Always. No matter how many miles we put on in a day he was behind the wheel. His favourite response when questioned about doing all of the driving on a trip was "If I'm too tired to drive, then everyone needs to get out for a stretch, a rest, or something to eat." He was right.

He had to fight hard not to sink into the depths of depression. Sometimes he failed, but he fought it and didn't give in for long.

Jack tends to have a negative personality. Usually seeing the dark and gloomy side of things, he is a true pessimist. I think part of it comes from the disease. Diabetes throws one thing after another at you. It is hard not to feel that life is bombarding you with more than you deserve, or can handle.

Often the symptoms are not readily visible and hard to describe, so the diabetic is sometimes looked at as being a malingerer or a hypochondriac, or, as my own father once cruelly said, "not good for much."

When someone has the ongoing and constantly changing effects of diabetes to contend with, depression, anger, and frustration are all part of the package he has been handed. Those who can fight those things and aim for a positive approach are to be admired.

Sometimes you just have to take things into your own hands and fight for your rights. Fight to get what you need.

IN SEARCH OF HEALTH CARE

We've had many challenges during our twenty-plus years of living with diabetes. One of the most tense, from my perspective, began when our family doctor left her practice. We suddenly found ourselves without a physician.

This was at a stage when Jack's health was particularly volatile. I was really worried. A look at his file at the doctor's revealed a hefty document, a good two inches or more thick. He needed consistency in his health care.

My first approach was to call every doctor in town to see if anyone was taking patients. None would even put Jack's name on a list. Next I called the medical association. They offered no help. Then I called the province's health officer. He suggested I put my name on a wait list. But, said I, no one will take his name on a waiting list.

As days passed with not even a glimmer of hope for finding a doctor, I decided this was one battle I was going to fight to win. I went to the media and told them my concerns about Jack's health and the ramifications of not having consistent medical care that took into account his varied problems. That resulted in a newspaper article and radio and television interviews. I decided to go to the top, so I began calling government officials, including the minister of health and the minister of transportation. (Jack's job depended on his driving. To continue driving he had to have a form filled in by his family physician. He didn't have a family physician. No doctor should be asked to offer such important life-changing opinions for a patient he or she doesn't know.)

I called the premier's office — in fact, I went through the government phone book and called everyone who had a job title that seemed to be even remotely connected with getting us a doctor. I didn't just call once and sit back and wait. I started every day with several phone calls to this group of people. I didn't often get to speak with the premier or ministers. But I'm sure my messages got through, even if was just a complaint that "that *?@#! woman who wants a doctor called again."

I joined forces with the local members of the public service union and as a result attended meetings with top government officials, which led to more media coverage.

Several times during my quest for a physician for Jack I was told he should go to a clinic. There are several evening clinics in town. They are a stop-gap between having a family physician and rushing to the hospital ER. I could just picture it. This man with a medical file several inches thick going to an unknown doctor who knows nothing about his pre-existing health challenges and prescribes some drug or changes a medication without referring to his records. Just the thought of it terrified me.

So by becoming a nuisance that would not go away I attained my goal.

One day the phone rang, and it was the chief medical officer (or some equally imposing title) calling. Dr. George Carruthers had agreed to take Jack as a patient. Not me, I was warned. He would only take Jack. Eventually, of course, the good doctor added me to his patient list as well.

It's a story too often told about people who don't have a doctor or a team of doctors who are specifically charged with looking after their diabetes care. How they survive is a mystery. Who prescribes their drugs? Who refers them to specialists? Who monitors their treatment?

These are the kinds of situations in which you have to take charge, to become your own advocate. Always think of the value you are putting on yourself. If you don't think you are worth fighting for, why should anyone else? Darn tooting, you're worth it.

There are other advocacy roles that need to be taken. Like any cause, diabetes needs people out there working for the general good.

GETTING INVOLVED RENEWS STRENGTH

DOH has a twelve-year-old daughter who is an insulin-dependent Type 1 diabetic. She is a role model for parents of children with diabetes. She gets involved at many levels and has become one of the very important people working as a volunteer.

"I try to help my daughter by being there for her. I make sure she attends her doctor's appointments and that she continues to learn more about caring for herself. I try not to feel sorry for her and I never encourage her to use her diabetes as an excuse to get out of chores or to not try new things. I try to teach her about the outside world and how she can do whatever she wants as long as she follows a few simple rules in terms of her care.

"I also got involved with a local parent support group and helped to organize special events for the children so that they could meet others living with diabetes. Rather than return to the paid workforce, I opted to stay home to ease the stress of our family and to be there at the school when my daughter was learning to test herself and do her own injections. I went on school trips when the teachers were afraid and attended her cross-country meets to ensure she wouldn't collapse due to a drop in blood sugar. I educated parents of her friends who invited her over and tried to treat her as a child first.

"Perhaps one of the most significant things that we did as a family was attend the Fourth Annual Friends for Life National Children with Diabetes Conference held in July 2003 at Disney World in Lake Buena Vista, Florida. About 1,500 people, representing thirty-six U.S. states and nine countries, including Canada, attended the four-day event. Included in the audience were over seven hundred children with diabetes and their siblings. Not only did my daughter get a chance to meet some celebrity role models with diabetes but she made a new friend while learning more about diabetes care. My husband and I also had a chance to listen to numerous experts in the field and realized that there were many people working towards a cure. We were not alone in our fight. That vacation, we learned to laugh again, knowing that our family had survived. We would highly recommend the experience to anyone with a child with diabetes. The trip was expensive but worth every penny.

"Since that conference, our family has had a renewed strength and we continue to look for ways to help our daughter. In November 2004, as part of National Diabetes Month, the local parent support group created an awareness campaign to help educate the public about the difference between Type 1 and Type 2 diabetes. At the same time, the children wrote letters to Santa asking him for a cure and created decorations for use on a Christmas tree promoting the Canadian Diabetes Association.

"When the Canadian Diabetes Association sent out a note asking for volunteers to tell their stories, I jumped at the opportunity and was pleased to hear so many others wanted to speak out as well. Now, after working with the direct marketing group in Toronto, our family's story will be part of a national holiday card campaign encouraging the public to help fund research and the work of the Canadian Diabetes Association.

"Working on these projects has given our family a sense of purpose, as we continue to live with my daughter's condition. Of course, there are many ways for families to get involved. We only wish we had the time to do more. Sometimes, you just have to run away. It's easy to burn out and not want to talk about diabetes anymore. That's when we pull back and try to live as normal a life as we can. After a rest, we find strength to speak out again."

She has advice to pass along to others who find themselves in a similar situation, dealing with diabetes.

"Do everything in your power to hang onto your family. You'll feel like you're in the middle of a storm, but in time the waters will calm down and peace will be restored. That doesn't mean the waves won't come crashing down again, but every time you're splashed in the face, take the experience and learn from it.

"As a freelance writer, back in July 2003, I had a chance to interview some celebrity role models with diabetes. One of them, Will Cross, was the first person with diabetes to walk to both the North and the South Poles. His advice: 'Use diabetes to your advantage.' In other words, you can sit there and feel sorry for yourself or you can get up, do something, and make it a better place. His goal was to prove that people with diabetes can do extraordinary things.

"So get involved. Start a support group. Become an advocate. Talk about diabetes. Share your knowledge. Tell your story. Educate the public. Lobby for more research monies. Canvas for such groups as the Canadian Diabetes Association or the Juvenile Diabetes Research Foundation. Ask questions. Look for answers. Make it a better place for people with diabetes."

Knowledge is power. Educating people passes knowledge to others and as a result gives the bearer of the message power. Power to make change, to gain understanding and sympathy to their goals. DOH is an active member of a local diabetes parent support group and since her daughter was diagnosed has written articles educating the public about diabetes. She worked with the Canadian Diabetes Association on a national holiday card fundraising campaign. One aspect of that campaign was, of course, promoting the project to the general public through a media release. I have included that release here, as it is an excellent example of how a support group can get its message out.

Sarnia/Lambton Diabetes Parent Support Group

MEDIA RELEASE

For Immediate Release:
Local Children and their Parents to Create Awareness of Type 1 Diabetes

TYPE 1? TYPE 2 DIABETES? IT'S ALL THE SAME, RIGHT? WRONG!

Local parents with children with Type 1 diabetes are getting tired of explaining the differences between the two major types of diabetes and are joining forces with their children to educate the public about how this medical condition is so misunderstood. They are launching an awareness campaign this month that will include a display in Lambton Mall November 17, 18 and 19, a special tree display at the Point Edward Charity Casino November 22 to January 10, and a letter-writing campaign to Santa and other prominent individuals.

"With November being Diabetes Awareness Month, we are determined to have our voices heard," said Karen Holland, spokesperson for the Sarnia/Lambton Diabetes Parent Support Group. "Our children did not get diabetes because of their poor eating habits nor their lack of exercise. That is what some people think because of the public health campaign to educate people on Type 2 diabetes. Rather our kids represent a small minority with a quiet voice. I think it would be easier if their condition would be named something different."

Approximately 10 percent of Canadians with diabetes have Type 1. This is a genetic predisposition now believed to be carried by many people but it takes a viral infection to trigger the autoimmune response that causes a person's body to attack his/her own insulin making cells. The islet cells on the pancreas are destroyed and because insulin can no longer be produced, the individual must receive it some other way.

"That does not mean taking a pill, or a watching one's diet," added Holland. "For the majority of the over 60 children (18 years and younger) with Type 1 diabetes in the Sarnia/Lambton area, it means taking over 1,460 blood sugar tests each a year. That's over 87,600 finger pokes in total for just 60 children. Try calculating those figures over their lifespan."

In addition, these children must receive insulin either via an insulin syringe or pen between two and six times a day or wear an insulin pump with site changes every three days.

"This is not an easy thing to live with," said Cathy Goossens, another parent from the group. "Sometimes it takes a long time to figure out a child's needs. Before trying the insulin pump, our daughter had six seizures. It frightened us so much I would set the alarm for three in the morning so that I could test her blood sugars to prevent her blood sugars from dropping too low."

Holland explained that insulin dosages are based on the blood sugar reading at the time. However, it is not a scientific formula and weather, stress, exercise, extra food and growth hormones can create havoc with the blood sugar levels. If a parent administers too much insulin, or if a child's blood sugars drop due to a number of reasons such as a skipped meal or extra exercise, there is an immediate danger. The child may feel shaky, get headaches and if left untreated the child could lose consciousness or have a seizure.

If a child does not receive enough insulin or decides to eat more than what he/she should, blood sugars can rise. Over a long period of time, high blood sugars can be the direct cause of a number of serious complications including heart disease, kidney disease, blindness and limb amputations.

"These are things the public does not see," said Holland, "and our children keep reminding us that diabetes is no picnic."

Some of the kids are writing letters to Santa asking him for a cure.

"I remember when I was little and I had to go to the hospital," wrote Hala Miller, a local child who has had Type 1 diabetes for over three years. "I was scared that I would never eat an apple again. So Santa I want toys but I don't. What I really want is a cure for diabetes."

Others are making decorations for a special tree that will be up at the local casino. A number of them are working on a display for the local mall.

"We may be a small voice," stressed Holland, "but we expect to grow louder."

Anyone interested in joining this local Diabetes Parent Support group may contact 542-7242.

For further information, contact:
Karen Holland
Spokesperson, Sarnia/Lambton Diabetes Parent Support Group
519-542-7242

There you have a darn good example of how a press release to the media can be used to help diabetics, and of how a group of parents took steps to be advocates for their children. This is also a good example of how a press release should be prepared to send to the media. Notice that it is a ready-to-read story, that it included newsworthy information, and that it has contact information at the bottom in case a reporter is assigned to follow up on the story.

It is important to recognize that the media (newspapers, radio, television) is usually very helpful in getting a message like this out. You need to have a good "angle" or a message with some news content, and remember that they do have a limit to how much time or space they can give you, so don't waste it or turn them off by demanding too much or by going to them without a good "story" or information to impart.

INFORMATION FLOW

Jack and I feel very fortunate in that we have the support of an excellent family physician, diabetes specialist, and diabetes educator. In fact, we have every confidence in the competent and caring medical professionals who are an important part of our lives. I sometimes feel that there is an important element of care missing for many people. Sometimes you encounter a physician or specialist who simply does not seem to acknowledge that diabetes should be considered when diagnosing or prescribing medication or treatment. This usually happens in an emergency or unexpected situation, but your diabetes can be overlooked in many situations.

In a perfect world all of your caregivers would sit around a table with you to discuss every facet of your health care before making any decisions. That is never going to happen. Our health care system just does not allow for it. No one has the time. Computerized systems are certainly helping to create an effective and efficient information flow, vastly improving the exchange of reports and histories, but even with the marvels of new technology it still comes down to the fact that you, the patient, need to take responsibility for making sure that everyone who is making decisions related to your health is aware of your diabetes and takes it into consideration. Printed information is best.

One thing you can do to this end is to become the carrier of important details. Let's suppose you are having tests done that send you to several different venues. Ask that all reports be sent to your family doctor. They may go to a specialist as well, but specifically ask that your family physician get a copy. Then, obtain a copy from your family doctor of the reports/results. You might not understand it, but what you can do is carry it with you when you go to the next appointment on your list. How many times has a doctor said, "I'll have to get a copy of that test"? So then you leave, make another appointment, and wait. It all takes time. If you have the test results in your possession and can hand them over, it not only saves time, but it also puts you there in the office while your doctor looks at them. He can ask questions while it is all fresh in his mind.

I also carry a list of all of the people involved in Jack's health care, with addresses and phone numbers, and have had occasion to hand it over to a doctor. I now have a binder at home with sheet protectors in it. I keep all things medical in it and have been known to put the whole binder in a carry bag and take it with us to hospitals and appointments. If we don't need it, no big deal, I just take it home again. But if we do need it, we are prepared.

CONTROL DURING SURGERY

Recently Jack was hospitalized for surgery. We supplied the surgeon with information about Jack's diabetes, including the fact that he is on the pump, during an office visit. Included in that information was the name of his oncologist in Saint John. The surgeon was not familiar with insulin pumps, so he followed up. We also typed out information about how to handle the pump, how to give extra insulin, and what Jack's base rates are. This was given to the charge nurse during Jack's pre-op session at the hospital. We met with the anesthesiologist to introduce him to the pump and again provided written information.

Finally we put Jack's pump into a strong, clean, self-sealing plastic bag, along with instructions for its use, my telephone number, and the number for the folks in charge over at Saint John Regional Hospital. That bag was pinned to the front of his hospital gown for the entire eleven days he was in the hospital, including during his surgery, when he left his pump on its regular setting. Other than going a little high on a few occasions his blood sugars remained stable.

Before the pump, sickness or surgery could trigger Jack to fluctuate all over the place, with some dangerous lows creating excitement among the nursing staff. This time, because he had the pump and because he stayed in control, his blood sugars did not add to the recovery time.

Both on his pre-admission test day and during his recovery Jack took the time to tell others what he was doing. Several times he did an impromptu "show and tell" session. As a result, the staff monitored his blood sugars by testing but left insulin adjustments to him. He did additional testing himself because he wasn't eating normally, allowing him to do adjustments as needed. It was a very positive experience.

The period following any trauma to the system, such as surgery or an injury, is one of those times when diabetics need to be monitored closely. Yet monitoring is difficult for nurses, who don't know your body and its normal reactions or patterns. You, or those around you, need to be aware and not just leave it to others to take over keeping your blood sugars in control.

In the course of writing this book I've talked to several people who did not feel they received proper or adequate medical care. It reinforced my belief that the patient needs to be a bit aggressive in being involved in his or her own care. We found every nurse but one (who just had a case of the grumps) to be terrific at the Queen Elizabeth Hospital in Charlottetown. Most importantly we found them to be interested in learning more about how Jack handled his insulin pump and very open to his asking questions and to asking some in return.

Although Jack had some complications that made for a few tense days, I believe that we had a positive experience with his most recent surgery because we made a real effort to communicate information about Jack's diabetes. We started in the surgeon's office and continued it every step of the way. I say "we" because I tend to be the documenter in the family. I keep the information, gather the things people need to know, type them out, and have it in hand. Jack is the communicator. He talks to people and will happily show them things when appropriate.

COSTLY IMPACT ON BUDGETS LARGE AND SMALL

Remember that I have been spouting off about diabetes having far-reaching effects that go beyond the individual. Consider this information obtained from the Internet.

The International Diabetes Federation says the World Health Organization (WHO) estimates that 4 to 5 percent of health budgets are spent on diabetes-related illnesses.

A person with diabetes incurs medical costs that are two to five times higher than those of a person without diabetes. This is due to more frequent medical visits, purchase of supplies and medication, and the higher likelihood of being admitted to a hospital.

Direct costs to people with diabetes and their families

These may be financial or non-financial in nature. The financial burden may be considerable if the individual or the family has to pay for medical care, drugs, insulin, and other supplies out of their own pocket.

Direct costs to health care system

These range from the relatively low cost items — primary care consultations and hospital outpatient episodes — to very high cost items, such as long hospital stays for the treatment of complications.

Action taken early in the course of diabetes is more beneficial in terms of quality of life and is more cost-effective, especially if this action can prevent hospital admission.

Indirect costs to society

While many people with diabetes continue to enjoy very productive working lives, both in paid employment and at home, some may not be able to continue working. Loss of productivity (resulting from disability, sickness, premature retirement, or premature death) is the most significant contributor to the indirect costs of diabetes.

Intangible costs

Intangible, or psychosocial, costs have the greatest impact on the lives of people with diabetes and their families, and include stress, pain, and anxiety. Life expectancy and quality of life can be significantly reduced by diabetes.

THE IMPORTANCE OF PROPER CARE

As this disease becomes increasingly widespread, everyone needs to become more aware and to take charge of how diabetes affects them and theirs. Diabetics need to control their disease and to work with whomever necessary to gain the best treatment so that the effects of diabetes are minimized.

The difference between diabetics who are getting good care and are in control and those who are not is a simple one for governments to put into perspective. Diabetics in control are able to maintain themselves, are contributing members of society. They work, they pay their way, and they don't stress the health care systems.

Diabetics who are not maintaining themselves will become users of the medical system. They will become dependent on society to support them as they slowly deteriorate. It's not a pretty picture. Not for the family who faces that future, not for the medical system that has to care for the individual, and not for the government and insurance companies who foot the medical bills.

There seems to be a very real gap in the system — both with the public reporting on diabetes through the media and with the government. There is a focus on prevention. Magazine articles, pamphlets, and all manner of materials are produced to try to prevent diabetes. At the other end of the scale our medical practitioners and health care providers, as well as the funding bodies, do their best to provide good patient care as the individual succumbs to one effect of the disease after another: blindness, heart attacks, kidney failure, bladder problems, circulation problems, debilitating fatigue — the list is long.

In the middle are the individuals who have diabetes and are struggling to maintain their health, to be self-supporting, to look after their families, and to be part of their community. To enjoy life, to be able to plan ahead to a good retirement and productive future are not impossible dreams for the diabetic. They need to get good health care, through availability of modern, up-to-date services, proper education, and resources to aid them to take responsibility for their own health.

Once they know what to do, most people will do it. But when you are sick with the disease and financially burdened by its costs it can become overwhelming. We find the cost of drugs and supplies, for example, to be increasingly difficult to cope with, and we have a good insurance that pays 80 percent. What do people who don't have that coverage do? Often they just can't test when they should or take the medication they are prescribed. A diagnosis of diabetes should not mean automatic relegation to the status of working poor, or, as a friend recently put it, the poorly retired.

TAKING CHARGE AND BECOMING AN ADVOCATE

It is unfortunately true that it does matter where you live when you have diabetes. If you live in a major centre with a large, accessible hospital that doesn't have long wait times, if you have a family physician and good diabetes education close at hand, count your blessings.

If you live in a rural area, a small town, or a have-not province, you have my heartfelt sympathy. You may well be facing the long-term effects of inadequate health care.

To my mind the most important factors in maintaining the best health possible as a diabetic are:

- good medical care with appropriate family physician and specialists;
- good education facilities that are readily available;

- good provincial and federal support with the cost of drugs, supplies, etc.;
- a good attitude towards self-management; and
- good support from family, friends, co-workers, and employers.

That said, the only people who can really dictate the diabetic's future health are the diabetic and her support group. That means taking charge of daily living and fighting for what you need. Sometimes it means doing research and taking on the government, the medical system, your employer, or your insurance company. Other times the biggest battle is with the patient herself.

Experts will tell you that diabetes care should be patient-centred and focused on self-management. Examples show again and again that this is the key. It must also be recognized that for the patient to do her job well, she needs the support behind her. In fact I searched the Web and found a summary from around the world that showed agreement that every diabetic should have:

- diabetes care that is standardized, equal, and readily available to all;
- initial and ongoing needs-based diabetes education, received in a timely manner;
- physicians who can effect timely diabetes management on an ongoing basis; and
- access to pharmaceuticals and medical devices that can improve quality of life.

None of this should depend on where you live or how much money you have!

BEWARE GOVERNMENT ACTIONS

People who care about their health and that of those around them really need to be aware of what governments are doing with health care. They need to be in the know and to be ready to step up and fight for quality care.

Sometimes things are masked by "announcements" or assurances that there will be no effect on the general population. Yeah, right! Frankly, people, it's time we got out there and started fighting for appropriate medical care. If we, people who are certain to need medical care, don't care enough to fight for it, then who will? And what right do we have to complain when it's not there if we sat back in apathy and didn't even bother to write a letter, to speak out, to voice our concerns?

Take Prince Edward Island, my home province. Consider these red flags that went up during the time I was researching this book.

1. Drug costs are increasing. The cost of insulin, for example, is subsidized, but the amount the patient pays has increased. It was stated that the extra cost to the individual would be less than $150 per year. In fact, when we calculated the cost to our household it was much higher.

2. A headline in the newspaper said, "Closure of N.B. hospital beds shouldn't affect Island patients." In June 2004 the New Brunswick government announced it was closing six hospitals and downsizing almost every remaining hospital, supposedly in an effort to create a more efficient system. So why, you ask, am I, a Prince Edward Islander, concerned that New Brunswick is losing three hundred hospital beds? The truth is that our health system relies on New Brunswick for some specialized health care. In our case, because Prince Edward Island does not have a diabetes specialist we have to travel to Saint John to access that care. If the hospital we deal with is now overburdened from within its own province, will that affect the availability of special care for Islanders? My guess would be yes.

3. Another area of concern to the diabetic is the long delays at emergency rooms, or, in a worst-case scenario, the closure of services at ERs. It doesn't sound important until you need one. Visit any ER and ask about the wait time. Then you will hope you never need one. These long waits have

led to some drastic measures. People who could walk in
now call an ambulance in hopes of faster service.

So what can we do? We must be advocates, act as watchdogs,
and speak up. We must join and support advocacy groups (numbers
count), we must speak up, join groups like Best Medicines Coalition
and the Canadian Diabetes Association, to get the message out that
we require and demand good health care.

Patients' voices need to be heard; if you, the patient, don't speak
out it just won't happen. It comes down to that same point. If you
don't care enough about your own health to fight for it, how can
you expect others to?

One more thing. Don't just complain to your medical support
team. Remember, the cutbacks and limitations are just as frustrating to
the doctors who are trying to get you services. It is the government
that holds the purse strings.

Volunteer. Work towards benefiting your health care system.
Stand up to be counted. Take responsibility.

FEAR OF "THE SYSTEM"

Sometimes rules and regulations become the enemy. This is a very
emotional issue that can lead to foolish decisions with regard to
overall health. Unfortunately, governments and others (such as
insurance companies), in trying to do the best for the common
good, can back people into a corner.

My example here is driving. I suspect each province differs, so
I'm going to create a scenario. Let's suppose that our pretend diabetic, we'll call him Dudley, realizes that his eyes have deteriorated
to the point that he is afraid he will lose his licence if his doctor
reports him. Now, Dudley feels like he is in control. He's careful. He's
never had an accident as the result of his eyes being less than they
used to be. Dudley is a family man. He has children to feed, clothe,
and care for. Dudley is scared. What if he goes to the doctor and the
doctor reports him as being unsafe to drive? He could lose his job.

He won't be able to find another one. He won't be able to take the kids where they want to go. He will, he thinks, be a lesser man.

So what does he do? He skips his eye appointment. He doesn't go to the doctor. He chooses to hide his condition. I know the temptation is there. Jack and I went through it. We were lucky that we didn't choose that route. We made the decision not to deny Jack medical treatment. But I will never deny that it was a hard decision at that time.

We saw people far less capable and fit to drive than Jack waltzing in and getting their driver's licence with no problem. Irresponsible people, people with very poor reaction time, people with heart problems, alcoholics, drug users — the list of people driving who shouldn't be is long. Yet diabetics and seniors seem to be targeted.

It's also a hard decision for physicians. They have been put in a position of throwing doctor-patient confidentiality out the window. It can't be easy, especially when they know that reporting a patient will affect the relationship they have with their patient.

I don't know what the answer is. Perhaps everyone should have to have mandatory checks independent of their personal medical professionals.

For the purpose of this book, I do urge diabetics to put their health first and not deny themselves the proper medical treatment because of fear of what might happen. Better you should maintain yourself in the best possible way for the longest period of time than risk it all for a few more months of driving a car.

Instead of battling the systems — or crying about it — put those energies into battling the disease.

SPEAK FOR YOURSELF

Listening to Oprah Winfrey today I heard her say something that really hit home. Although I didn't get the exact quote, the gist of what she said is "The courage to speak your own truth helps not only yourself, but someone else — each time you do it."

It is so true. There are times when you just have to say, "I'm sorry, that is not acceptable. I am a diabetic and I need _____ [fill in the blank]." When you do that you not only make people aware of your needs and rights as a diabetic but also pave the way for those who follow.

You might be speaking to a waitress who is ignoring you when you need juice to counteract a low blood sugar episode.

You might be speaking to a host at a dinner party that is running late.

You might be heading out for a walk when everyone wants you to veg out, eat chips, and watch television.

You might be trying to make a doctor's appointment for something you feel is urgent and being told there is a six-week wait.

You might simply need a prescription filled today.

The point is you need to take charge, and the best way to begin is with simple things. Taking charge of your own health often begins with a small step triggered by something you read or hear. There are three steps here:

1. Accept responsibility and become action oriented.
2. Have an open mind and be receptive to learning from the experiences of others.
3. Never hesitate to educate those you come into contact with.

The last point is as important as the first two. For example, many feel that all a diabetic has to do to stay healthy is inject insulin. We all know that insulin is a therapy; it is not a cure. It is up to us to tell people that diabetics must manage everything they do and eat every day.

Taking charge means many things. Advocacy, certainly. It also means managing so that you control your life and live up to your own ideals. The following story is a great way to end this chapter. This little girl is a role model we can all follow.

TAYLOR'S STORY

Pamela J. Findlay is one proud mom in Vancouver, British Columbia, who wrote to share her daughter's story. Taylor has Type 1 diabetes.

"My daughter Taylor was diagnosed January 15, 2001. Three days prior to her sixth birthday. The information we received at that time regarding how profoundly our lives were about to change was overwhelming to say the least. In an attempt to keep focused on the point of this story, I won't go into the day-to-day reality that followed the diagnosis.

"As Halloween was approaching that year, my husband and I weren't sure how to handle it. Taylor was just getting used to her two needles per day, and up to eight blood tests. She had endured a myriad of birthday parties with cake and goodies being eaten all around her, and rarely complained.

"Two weeks before Halloween, Taylor approached her father and me with a 'proposal.' She wanted to dress up and go out for Halloween, but knew she couldn't eat the candy. She proposed to 'sell' the candy back to us for a sum of $40. We thought the amount was very high, but agreed nonetheless. With the $40 she bought herself a toy, but the issue still remained, what do we do with the candy?

"Taylor suggested we donate it to the Pediatric Ward of Royal Columbian Hospital (where she stayed when she was diagnosed). What a great idea! The kids who couldn't go out for Halloween due to injury or illness could still have candy.

"This idea has blossomed since that Halloween three years ago. Taylor still donates her candy (although we came to an agreement for a lesser amount), but she also donates other things through the year as well. We clean out her room of stuffed animals and movies that she no longer watches and she donates those to the ward as well. She has donated so many stuffed animals that Pediatrics now sends a stuffed animal home with each patient admitted. We won't be able to keep them in stuffed animals indefinitely, but we are so proud of what we have been able to provide thus far.

"Her pediatrician also calls her from time to time and asks if she would mind talking to a newly diagnosed child, and if I would speak with the parents. This seems to have given some sense of comfort to those families overwhelmed by an uncertain future.

"There it is. In no circumstance is living with Type 1 diabetes a 'good thing,' nor is it easy for a child. It is a series of blood tests, needles and/or food dispensed every two hours, 24 hours a day. Diabetes never takes a holiday, and although we are optimistic for a cure, the reality is there is no cure. That being said, this disease has been inflicted on my daughter, and I couldn't be more proud of how she's handling it.

"I am biased where Taylor is concerned. I do think she is an inspiration. She certainly inspires me."

We agree. Taylor is an inspiration! Not only did she find a way to compensate herself for not having all that candy, but she also helps others, and by talking to other newly diagnosed children and their parents she has taken the role of generous contributor to others to a new, higher level. Taylor and her family are truly taking charge, taking control, and becoming true advocates.

CHAPTER 8

Pumping to Quality of Life

January 3, 2003

Things took an amazing turn towards the normal in our household today. It's January. It's cold. The ground is covered with snow, and ice covers the driveway. It's dark. A storm is pending. And — here is the normal part — Jack has been outside for hours, fixing the brakes on our old Jetta. And I have been out there with him, holding the light.

You see, in the past Jack could be counted on to be doing something major — and with consequences if it didn't get finished — in the cold, dark days of winter. Take the Jetta, for instance. Today our van was towed to the repair shop with possible major problems, so the Jetta is our only mode of transportation. This storm that is coming is bringing major snow and probably high winds. Can't you just picture it — the job half done, tools and car bits all over the driveway buried until the next thaw. If that happens everything will be wrecked by rust or lost or something equally dramatic. So there is some urgency to get it done.

The brake fix didn't go smoothly — it's an old car with equally old rusted, worn wheels to deal with — but it did go.

He didn't blow up, although he did mutter a bit — but justifiable muttering at seized bolts and things like that. He kept at it and got it done. His only grousing revolved around stiff joints — getting up and down is harder these days — and being cold.

Later, doing the dishes to get his hands warmed, the man was fairly brimming over.

"Six weeks ago, I couldn't have thought about doing that, let alone doing it and feeling good. I didn't have the strength or the energy. I really didn't feel like I was going to live," he marvelled.

Even more incredible: after a mandatory blood check and resulting chocolate treat because he was "a little low," he whistled his way to his workshop to do another portion of a project he's been working on (a bench with a flip-up lid to hold the recyclables and provide a place to sit while we put our boots on). Again, something he could not have done before the big change.

And, that evening, even though I had taken the dog for a walk to save Jack from having to go out in the cold again he up and took her around the block again.

Amazing! So what brought about this change?

Jack was six weeks into being an insulin pump user. Six incredible weeks of rediscovering life, of eating foods that had been forbidden for years, of learning to move off the clock a little at a time. It's hard to allow yourself to break from that rigid "Thou shall eat at 7:00 a.m., noon, and 5:30 p.m. or be in trouble" routine.

Six weeks of getting back a quality of life we had forgotten about.

So, how did this all come about? A brief recap. Jack had heard about insulin pumps while watching golf on television. We began researching them and after two years were referred to Dr. John Dornan at Saint John Regional Hospital. After an assessment Jack was approved as a likely pump candidate. We were told to acquire a pump, learn carb counting, and then go back for pump startup.

Since one of the biggest areas of concern for us was the uncertainty of each step ahead of us, the fear of the unknown, I want to give you a bit of a step-by-step accounting of what took place with the pump. So many people ask about the details, so here they are. Each situation, each individual, each hospital, each doctor will vary in how things are done and have their own way of doing things, but this will give you an idea.

Our first appointment, for evaluation, required a day at the hospital in Saint John. Because the appointment was early we went the day before and stayed in a hotel for the night. It is a five- to six-hour drive for us to Saint John.

Saint John Regional Hospital has one of the slickest, smoothest systems I have ever encountered. You check in with one of several people right in the lobby — there is no question of where to go. They take your insurance and medical coverage information, tap away on their computer keyboard, and then send you off with directions for where to go and when to be there. It is a very welcoming and easy beginning to your hospital experience.

From the lobby it's off to the appropriate waiting room. As you arrive your information is being printed out at the reception desk. Before many minutes we were called into an office where a doctor asked what seemed like hundreds of questions, writing everything down in great detail. After about half an hour he said he didn't think Jack needed an insulin pump, but the final decision lay with Dr. John Dornan. Taking the paper with him he left to confer with Dr. Dornan.

Our hopes plunged during those few minutes we waited. We tried to stay cheerful, to boost each other up, but it was hard. We had been grasping at the idea of a pump making life better like a drowning man reaching for a rope.

When Dr. Dornan walked in he spent a minute or two looking over the papers, asked Jack a number of questions, and then turned to the first doctor and said, "I have to disagree with you. I think Jack is an excellent candidate for pump therapy."

He then explained the procedure, sent Jack for blood tests, and referred us to the Diabetes Education Centre within the hospital. There we met Linda Graham, department manager, and her team. Again we were given information such as where to obtain a pump, appointments were set, and so on. Again it was very friendly and caring. For Jack and I it was so wonderful to be in the presence of these cheerful, positive people.

We had already done some research and went through the process of obtaining our pump, a D-TRONplus from Disetronic. That step is detailed in chapter six. If you want to put things into sequence, refer back to the beginning of chapter six and "insert here." I'm jumping ahead to our return to Saint John for pump startup.

What an exciting time. We were eager, apprehensive, nervous. We had been told to report in on Monday morning and expect to be there for about five days. Accommodation was a bit of an issue for us because of the cost. Although our province has good medical coverage, and we have medical insurance carried over from Jack's job, there is nothing to help defray costs such as those related to travelling for medical treatment. Those costs can be devastating for families.

At first we thought Jack would be hospitalized. He had been when he went on insulin injections years before. But, no, we were told we could monitor ourselves. Scary thought, being alone overnight with this new apparatus to contend with.

Since money was an issue we looked at the outpatient housing through the hospital. That was inexpensive for Jack, but I could not stay with him and would have to pay for my own accommodation at a hotel. We had also been told that someone should be with him during the night to help with monitoring.

The representative from our pump manufacturer had a policy of being with her clients to help with startup, so we checked into the same hotel she was at, the Howard Johnson on Main Street in Saint John, which gives a special rate to those receiving treatment at the hospital. The pump company rep was in the room beside ours, and across the hall were a mother and her daughter, who was also going to start pumping. We met the evening before Jack's appointment at the hospital and went out to supper together. It was a good thing that reinforced my belief that a team approach is best. We felt that team support even before we got to the hospital.

Prior to going to Saint John Jack had obtained his pump and practised coding it, changing insulin, and replacing batteries — everything except actually hooking it up to his body. Again the pump rep had given us demonstrations and helped Jack familiarize himself with the pump.

On arrival at the hospital, we went to the Diabetes Education Centre, where Jack was given a complete run-through on pump therapy, use of his pump, detailed step-by-step demonstrations, how to monitor it, and finally how to hook himself up to this new, life-giving apparatus. It seemed like no time before he was connected and clipping the pump onto his belt. (The pump is connected to an insert, or catheter, in his belly by a fine tube. It's flexible, easy to do, and, he says, comfortable.) We were told to go have something to eat and take a walk. We checked back in just to make sure things were okay, and then we were on our own.

We had instructions for the evening: how to count our meal and how to monitor Jack's blood. We were told to set the alarm so that we could check that things were going well during the night. We were helped with that the first night because Melany, the pump representative, came over to our room at 3:00 a.m. to make sure we were okay, something she also did for the mother and daughter across the hall. Everything was fine.

One of Jack's biggest concerns that first night was what to do with the pump when he was in bed. There is a natural fear of lying on it, damaging it, getting tangled in the tubing, or even of accidentally pulling the insertion site out. Everyone has to figure out what works best for him. Much of the decision depends on your sleeping habits. Jack started with a soft pouch hung around his neck and tucked inside his T-shirt. That works for him because he never sleeps on his stomach.

During the day he keeps his pump in a leather holder with loops that his belt slips through. It has clear plastic widows that allow him to flip the holder down so that he can easily see the screen and access the control buttons. Or, when puts on his "comfies" (a.k.a. gym pants) for lounging in front of the TV, he slips it into the pocket. When you purchase a pump you will be given several options for wearing it: pouches, clips, or straps.

Each day we checked in to the hospital to make sure things were going as they should, then had the rest of the day free — with instructions to walk, to be active, and to monitor well. On the third day Jack did a site change and had no problems. He amazed me with his "just do it" approach to all of these new things. He had

some nervous moments, but they never lasted long. He had practised with the pump until he felt very familiar with it. Any questions
that came up could be answered by referring to the detailed
instruction manual and information given to us.

Although Jack has never become at ease working with his
home computer, he was determined to get comfortable with the
pump. In the beginning I often read the instructions out loud so
that he could follow along, step by step. We still use that technique
for something we haven't done for a while, such as time changes,
or if he gets an unfamiliar error message.

By tackling it like that he soon gained confidence and felt at
ease with the pump.

On the fourth day we were given the okay to head home. Those
four days in Saint John for startup were like a mini vacation. We
explored the city, visited the farmers' market and museums, went
for drives in the country, and tried out new restaurants.

On the way home we were hit anew by the freedom we now had.
No need to panic if we were still a few miles from our favourite restaurant at lunchtime. Jack could basically eat what he wanted as long as
he counted the carbs accurately — what a treat. Although he doesn't
abuse this privilege and is still very aware of restricting his sugars and
fats and of eating as healthy as he can, he now can occasionally have
those things that were forbidden before. Somehow, now that he
knows he can have them he doesn't get the intense cravings he used
to. More often than not he turns down desserts, fried foods, and such.

But now it's his decision. It isn't forced on him! Wonderful how
liberating that simple fact is.

One thing I would like to point out for anyone who is apprehensive about going on the pump: there were some similarities between
Jack's starting on the pump and his start on insulin years before. The
apprehension, the uncertainty about being able to do the injections,
compares to learning how to give those first injections using the
pump. It's hard at first but quickly becomes part of daily routine.

I will never forget when he started on insulin injections. After a
couple of days in the hospital they gave him a day pass and told us
to go out for a good, brisk walk. He felt so good he leapt into the air

and clicked his heels to the side, just like a dancer in a movie. We laughed like a couple of giddy kids — because he could. We're older now. He had a lot of recovering to do; he was not as agile and spry, so the leaping part wasn't there, but the euphoria of feeling so much better physically and mentally certainly was.

Increased energy, decreased mood swings, less danger of overnight hypoglycemia, prevention of exercise-related low blood sugar reactions, the freedom to sleep late or go out to a late evening dinner on the spur of the moment, the personal power of feeling in control all added up to an improved outlook on life. In fact, the phrase "It's a wonderful life" kept popping into my head.

Pumps are expensive, and so are the supplies you will need. But both Jack and I are adamant in saying we would sell our house and all our possessions to keep him on the pump. What good are things if you can't enjoy them? When you weigh the cost against the quality of life, the ability to work, your eyesight, and your health, the scales surely do tip in favour of pumping.

It should be noted that some of the information about pumps, terms and such, comes from Disetronic, a company that makes insulin pumps. Jack uses a D-TRONplus from Disetronic, so that is the one we are familiar with. There are other pumps on the market, and you should explore them all before making your decision. You will need to become familiar with the one you select.

INSULIN PUMPS — WHAT ARE THEY?

Insulin pumps are marvellous little mechanical devices that make life so much easier and can amaze you with the great benefits they bring in a small package.

Computerized and programmable, they help diabetics by delivering fast-acting insulin, known as basal insulin, in very small precise amounts twenty-four hours a day. This continuous stream of insulin deals with your metabolic needs. Extra doses or larger amounts of insulin, keyed in to compensate for a meal or snack, are known as boluses. The insulin pump replaces insulin injections.

The pump delivers fast-acting insulin via a plastic catheter to an infusion set or small needle inserted through the skin. Minute doses are delivered automatically and accurately for gradual absorption into the bloodstream. Generally the site of insulin delivery is changed every third day. Much better than several injections per day.

It is important to remember than an insulin pump is a tool that you operate. It cannot measure or control blood sugars on its own. It must be programmed by you. You must do frequent blood sugar monitoring to gather the information needed to program effectively.

The actual amounts of insulin delivered are predetermined by the diabetic and his medical team. There are a variety of programming options that allow you to adjust dosages to fit any situation.

On the pump, you can live with spontaneity again: eat when you wish and go where you want, when you want. You can easily adjust to any situation. For example, in the summer Jack heads out early each morning for eighteen holes of golf. This increased activity is easily handled by adjusting insulin, testing his blood, and taking along an extra snack. He can even enjoy the occasional beer on a hot day.

Pumps are about the size of a deck of cards and must remain with a person at all times. They can be clipped to a belt, hung from a bra or around your neck, strapped to an arm or leg, or slipped into sewn pouches in your clothing. They can be hidden beneath clothing or proudly displayed for all to see. They weigh only a few ounces.

Pumps also come with built-in safety features such as alarms to let you know, for example, when the batteries are low or a mandatory inspection is required. They also let you know when insulin in getting low and they have key locks to avoid accidental activation or change and can be linked up with your personal computer.

The problem of bedtime pumping is easily resolved. The pump just keeps on doing whatever you programmed it to do. You can clip it to your nightwear, slip it under your pillow, or sew a pocket somewhere convenient. If romance is in the making, just lay the pump out of the way or disconnect for a while. If the thought of the pump interfering or creating the wrong image during sexual interludes even enters your mind, just think of this — without the pump, would you have the desire, the will, or the performance ability?

Remember that pumps should enhance your lifestyle by making it easier and safer for you to be active and flexible in your routines.

To my mind the key to successful pumping is working with your health care team: your doctor, who works with you to determine your unique therapy routine, and the pump supplier, who provides the support you need to carry out that prescribed treatment. Then take advantage of the power it gives you to get active. Activity and good health go together.

GET COMMITTED

Making the move to become a pumper is like getting married. Both a pump and a marriage require commitment and ongoing care and dedication to be successful.

- Test your blood sugars regularly, perhaps more often than in the past.
- Learn how to operate your pump and be familiar with every step needed to maintain your health.
- Be aware of what you eat, count the carbohydrates, work out the bolus amounts, and take them.
- Decrease insulin when you are very active.
- Learn to think like a pancreas.
- Maintain your supplies.
- Change your site as recommended.
- Keep your site and equipment clean to avoid infection.
- Exercise and be active.
- Accept that you must eat right — just as everyone else does.
- Maintain your visits to your family physician and medical caregiving professionals so that you are monitored and kept on track.

This seems like a long list, but most of it is already part of every diabetic's life, and all of it becomes simple with a little practice.

PUMPING TECHNOLOGY

Pumpers use a language of their own. The world of pumping is full of terms that they, medical professionals, and pump suppliers use. It's not complicated and it helps explain the pump.

Basal rate or basal insulin

A continuous twenty-four-hour delivery of insulin that matches background insulin need. These small regular releases of insulin imitate the natural action of the pancreas. The rate of insulin delivery you need is set by your physician and varies from person to person. When the basal rate is correctly set, the blood sugar does not rise or fall during periods in which the pump user is not eating. Basal rates are usually given as units per hour (u/hr), which are delivered in increments every few minutes.

Carb bolus

A spurt of insulin delivered quickly to match carbohydrates in a meal or snack. Again, the amount, or number of units of insulin, taken for the grams of carbohydrates is determined by your doctor.

High blood sugar bolus

A spurt of insulin delivered quickly to bring high blood sugar back to normal.

Infusion set

The hub, catheter, and insertion set that connect the pump to your body.

Insertion set

The part of the infusion set inserted through the skin. It may be a fine metal needle or a larger metal needle that is removed to leave a small catheter.

Catheter

The plastic tube through which insulin is delivered to the body, via the insertion set.

One of the things to look into when choosing a pump is the cost. Each pump company should be able to give you costs to purchase the pump as well as an estimate of monthly costs for operation. They will also have various payment options. Most pump suppliers are familiar with dealing with various insurance companies and will work with you to ensure that you obtain your entitled insurance coverage.

There are many questions you should ask:

- How much does it cost to purchase the pump?
- How much do monthly supplies cost, and how do I obtain them?
- What are the details of the return policy?
- What kind of warranty does the manufacturer offer?
- What happens if there is a pump failure?
- What kind of support is there for startup, training, and in case of questions or problems?
- How will the company work with me to get a system that is right for me?

The issue of what happens when a pump fails is an important one. You need to know whether there are spare pumps available and how long it will take to get one, how long the repair will take, and any costs involved for the repair work or for shipping. In our case the company we deal with provides a backup pump. The pump purchase included two pumps: one to use and one to keep as a backup in case of accident, a mechanical problem, or mandatory inspection. When you do not have a pump at hand you will need to go back to injecting insulin, so you also need to get your doctor to write down what your injection routine should be in case of pump failure. It's hard to remember those old dosages once you get on your pump.

PM's story demonstrates the improved quality of life possible with the insulin pump but also the determination and attention to detail needed to determine exactly what works for you.

ONE PUMPER'S STORY

PM, a Type 1 diabetic, is a thirty-five-year-old resident of Moncton, New Brunswick. She has been treated with diet, pills, and insulin, which she has been on for thirty-two years.

"I had been interested in the idea of an insulin pump ever since I was a kid when I first started reading about them in the *Diabetes Dialogue* [the magazine published by the Canadian Diabetes Association]. At that time there were no places near me where one could get the supplies or pumps and they seemed very, very expensive, big and not popular in the Moncton area.

"A few years ago I was performing in a dinner theatre at my church and was heard saying 'eating supper courses every half-hour will not work with my diabetes and insulin I need to take' (with an insulin pen/syringe at that time). A nurse, also in the choir, told me I should consider getting an insulin pump that seem to be available at this time.

"So, when I had an appointment to see my endocrinologist that June after a blood test indicating my HBA1C was too low (6.3) (preferred 6.8, 6.9, 7.0) Dr. M brought up the idea of the insulin pump. I told her how the nurse mentioned it to me and how it can be set to give insulin at different times to look after the lows and highs, fats.... I ended up ordering it right away and checking with my teacher's insurance to see if they would pay. It paid 80 percent. Within a month it was delivered.

"At first it was a hassle getting used to it, as when I was first hooked up to it at the end of my summer holidays, work was just starting again (I began teaching in a new school closer to home). The first insertion set did not work for me (Quick set), as I was a little too active for it. I switched to the Silhouette, which was sturdier and more anchored. I found the 508 Medtronic pump too big and bulky in September 2002. Things turned for the better in January 2003 when I was able to trade for the smaller paradigm Medtronic pump and switched to the Silhouette insertion set.

"After these changes my life quality started changing for the better. My face cleared up. No more breakouts, which I figured out were caused by eating something to bring my sugars up fast causing a reaction. My blood sugar levels were more stable during the night. No highs or lows happened as much overnight. I could eat pizza and pasta by setting the dual wave option on the pump and not have my sugars spike at 3:30 or 4:00 in the morning if I punched in the right amount of insulin.

"I had more energy at work and could think better and get my lesson plans done up much faster for the next day after the students left. I did not have the mood swings or emotional ups and downs I found I experienced especially when my period began. The biggest thing my mom noticed and my siblings, when they were home for a visit, was my confidence level, common sense advice and ability to shrug off things that were bothering me. Also, the biggest joy in my life was a meeting a man whom I started going out with that I used to know as a teenager working at McDonald's. We ended up getting married this past summer in July. He considers me as normal and more put together than women he knew who did not have diabetes! Married life is going well.

"I still get some high blood sugars and lows due to changes in routines, being busy (not enough hours in the day), stress, colds, menstruating, and cold weather (sugars go up) and hot humid weather (sugars drop). I did have surgery on my right eye back in 1998 after a lot of stress (death in family of Dad, laid off from work due to low student enrollment in school, sister separating from husband and not knowing where she was, buying own home after getting back to work teaching), ups and downs using insulin syringes, pressure on eye. Luckily I had a great eye doctor who did great laser treatment. My right eye lost a bit of sight but my left eye is as good as new.

"I find the pump is not a cure but it sure cuts down on the amount of things I need to think about in the run of a day. I am thankful for a supportive husband and family members over the years. I think all insulin diabetics should be on a pump. They should not look at it as being a guinea pig to try it out. I look forward to having a blood sugar monitoring device/insulin pump as an implant if the pancreatic cell implants do not work out.

"I am not sure if children are in the picture for my husband and I, as I do not want eye problems to return due to pressure. My diabetes and age (thirty-five) make having kids a difficult decision. Monitoring my blood sugars at work is difficult and I know my sugars will go up and down if I were expecting. Blood sugars need to be treated seven to nine times a day if one is pregnant. We'll see where we are in a year's time."

If you are considering a change to insulin pumping, you can find information about it through your physician, at the offices of the Canadian Diabetes Association, or by referring to the Internet.

You can also contact Insulin Pumpers Canada. This federally incorporated, not-for-profit, volunteer organization began as a local support group for people who were using or considering insulin pump therapy for themselves or their children. Their mission is to promote insulin pump therapy and help users optimize its benefits by providing support, education, information, and advocacy for people with diabetes, their families, health care professionals, and the general public.

In their brochure they say that what they are evolving into is directed by the visions of members. Membership is free. Here is a wee excerpt from their brochure:

> Pumps allow the user to participate more normally and more safely in daily activities. "Pumpers" can be any age (some are as young as new born babies)! Pumps may help delay the disabling and deadly long term effects of Diabetes.
>
> Insulin Pump Therapy is highly technical. The user must be highly educated on the technical, medical and bio-mechanical aspects of this therapy.
>
> We seek to fill the void between what medical professionals can do for people with Insulin Dependent Diabetes and what people who use insulin pumps require in order to optimize their

blood glucose control and quality of life by effectively utilizing the insulin pump.

Divisions or Affiliates of Insulin Pumpers Canada are located in several parts of Canada offering support and education at the local or regional levels. Want to start a pumpers group in your area? Contact us....

One of the things I think is so important about this group is that they provide support for parents of children who are considering and/or using insulin pumps. They raise the profile of pumping, provide support and knowledge, and since they are not affiliated with any pump company they are an excellent source of information.

It is also important to acknowledge their role as advocates. As this book is coming into being a bill has been introduced in Ontario to have OHIP cover the cost of insulin pumps and supplies; the website contains this and much more information. It contains provincial issues, references to good reading material, all manner of things. It even links to "Pump Expeditions," a simulation game to help adults and kids experience what life would be like on an insulin pump provided by Medtronic MiniMed, links to the four pump suppliers in Canada and other international pumpers organizations. Check it out. To contact them:

Insulin Pumpers Canada
National Office
P.O. Box 324
Lower Sackville, NS
B4C 2T2

Or visit their website at http://www.insulin-pumpers.ca.

CHILDREN AND PUMPING

Other than relating the personal experiences of diabetics who contributed their stories to this book I have not addressed the issue of children with diabetes. That is with reason. I personally have no experience in this area so cannot even consider writing about it. I will, however, pass along a few comments Dr. Gary Costain made when speaking at a meeting of the Prince Edward Island chapter of the Canadian Diabetes Association in Charlottetown.

"It is most important to let them live and develop as normally as possible for obvious reasons. It is very easy to get overprotective. It's not always easy, but let kids make own decisions in terms of what they want."

If, for example, you are considering an insulin pump for your child, he says, the time for kids to go on pumps is when they are ready psychologically. His other words of wisdom:

- Trying to convince kids to do the right thing can alienate them.
- Be honest about diabetes.
- Share information and educate their peers.
- Don't underestimate your kids.
- If people are open with it everyone will be happier.

Of the pump he said: "I think we have so many tools now. Our standard of care should be at least four injections a day. We can get pretty good control with four times a day. However, there is a better chance of getting people to target with a pump." Although a lot of people want islet cell transplants that lead to being put on immune support (immune suppressive drugs), he says, "The best option we have now is probably the insulin pump if doing insulin four times a day."

He confirmed that the main problem with the insulin pump is the cost. Insurance companies require pre-approval, and some give people a hard time, but if they persist the insurance companies will approve them. He suggested that those interested in the pump should use the people who act as advocates for patients with insurance companies. Your doctor should be able to link you with them.

A final note from this meeting was to beware of so-called miracle cures that are not coming through regular medical professionals.

"If something is good, a cure, a miracle medicine," said Dr. Costain, "the news will get out."

Since no chapter on pumping would be complete without addressing children, I was very pleased when MH of Ontario shared the following story of her son's experience with pumping.

THERE IS NOTHING THAT MCKENZIE CAN'T DO!

"In April 2001 the life of our young son was changed forever, as was the life and dynamics of our family.

"McKenzie was diagnosed just before his tenth birthday with Type 1 (insulin-dependent) diabetes. There is no history in our family of diabetes so this diagnosis came as a shock but not as a complete surprise.

"In looking back, McKenzie had displayed uncharacteristic mood swings and had occasionally complained that his eyes were sore. It wasn't until returning from a vacation by car that I noticed McKenzie was urinating too frequently. During this time I attributed it to the minor cold he had but mother's intuition nagged me to take him to the doctor's office.

"During the doctor's visit I was reassured that everything was fine with McKenzie but I was not comfortable with this and insisted that he be tested for diabetes. While I didn't know a lot about diabetes at that time I had read enough to know what some of the symptom were.

"My fears were confirmed just days before Easter in 2001, at which time I went from not knowing much about diabetes to getting my hands on all I could read about this chronic illness in an attempt to help my son cope with his/our new life challenge. Talk about being on a steep learning curve and at the same time trying to maintain some semblance of normality in an already very busy household.

"Our life was suddenly and constantly regulated by the time of the clock and food became an enemy of sorts that required measuring and counting not to mention the pain that was measured by the five injections of insulin a day. How we longed for those carefree days when food was a joy and didn't require any pain associated with it or much thinking. How I longed as a mother to be able to take this chronic illness away from my son and keep it myself.

"In my search for treatment options I was told about insulin pump therapy.

"McKenzie started on his insulin pump in February 2002 and with it his quality of life and his ability to have direct control over his diabetes was given back to him.

"While the initiation of insulin pump therapy is time consuming and a whole new learning experience we embraced this opportunity to find a way that would allow McKenzie to live in better harmony with his chronic illness.

"Insulin pump therapy has allowed McKenzie for the most part to live a life parallel to when he did not have diabetes. McKenzie has taken on the responsibility with my help to manage his diabetes. He has proven himself to be a very capable and responsible person who still continues to amaze me.

"Insulin pumps come with different built-in controls that allow a parent to let their children have no or ever-increasing responsibility for the operation of their insulin pump.

"Insulin pump therapy allows McKenzie to do all the things that most people do without much thought like eating when they want, what they want or not eating at all.

"Sleeping in, sleeping over, playing all types of sports like squash, soccer or just bouncing on the trampoline. There is nothing that McKenzie can't do!

"Insulin pump therapy had such a huge impact on our lives that I felt compelled to work for an insulin pump company to help people like ourselves make a smooth transition to insulin pump therapy and to a better quality of life.

"I know I have the best job in the world and have learned all of the positive things about diabetes through the many friends I have met who have shared their diabetes with me.

"I urge anyone interested in finding out more about insulin pump therapy to visit www.insulin-pumpers.ca."

And so, we come to the end. I intentionally left this chapter to the end because I wanted to end this book on a positive note. I feel a bit like a preacher at this point, always stressing the "take charge, take control, be responsible" angle. I do think it is important, not only to maintaining the best physical health but also to keeping the mind in good order.

Diabetes is a terrible disease. Yet, think of this. At least with diabetes, you, the patient, you, the family member or friend, can do something to help yourself. Any time you are heading for a pity party, head instead for a hospital or a facility for those with special needs or a rehabilitation institute. Look at the battles others face. When you put it in perspective, controlling your eating, getting some exercise, taking pills, living by the clock, even giving yourself a needle is nothing compared to what some people face every day. Nothing.

Go forward, my friends, with a positive attitude and a determination to live the best you can every day. Take time to savour what is around you. There is beauty and joy everywhere. Take pleasure in the small things. Savour your small victories. Have a good day. Rejoice in it.

And always remember that knowledge is power that takes on even more strength when combined with action.

FOR MORE INFORMATION

The following organizations are excellent sources of information ranging from helpful hints for daily living to updates on new research and special conferences, events, and activities:

Canadian Diabetes Association
Website: www.diabetes.ca
Email: info@diabetes.ca
Phone: 416-363-0177 or 1-800-BANTING (1-800-226-8464)
Fax: 416-408-7117

Check your local telephone directory to find a branch office near you.

Canadian Health Network
Website: www.canadian-health-network.ca

This is a website of the Public Heath Agency of Canada.
Check your local government listings for contact information.

Canadian Pensioners Concerned
Website: www.canpension.ca.
Email: info@canpension.ca
Phone: 416-368-5222 or 1-888-822-6750
Fax: 416-368-0443

Diabetes Online
Website: www.diabetes.gc.ca
Email: EICDPD-DPIPMMC@phac-aspc.gc.ca

This is a website of the Public Heath Agency of Canada.
Check your local government listings for contact information.

Disetronic Medical Systems, Inc.
Website: www.Disetronic-usa.com
Phone: 1-800-280-7801
For Canadian information email:
melany.hellstern@disetronic-usa.com

Juvenile Diabetes Foundation Canada
Website: www.jdrd.ca
Email: general@jdrd.ca
Phone: 905-944-8700 or 1-877-CURE-533
Fax: 905-944-0800

Meditronic MiniMed (Insulin Pumps)
Website: www.minimed.com
For Canadian sales reps in your area phone:
1-800-284-4416.

American Diabetes Association
Website: www.diabetes.org
Email: AskADA@diabetes.org
Phone: 1-800-DIABETES (1-800-342-2383)

OTHER USEFUL WEBSITES:

Insulin Pumpers Canada.
Website: www.insulin-pumpers.ca

International Diabetes Federation
Website: www.idf.org

Dictionary of Diabetes Terminology
Website: www.diabetes.org/diabetesdictionary.jsp

SPECIAL THANKS TO:

Tracey Allen, Dan Amero, Helen Bates, Anne Choi, Dr. Gary Costain, Aileen Eaton, Pamela J. Findlay, Kerry Fry, Westen Fry, Jean Gamble, Debbie Gamble-Arsenault, Helen Grant, Cheryl Keddy, Patricia Kelly, Janet MacDonald, Barbara McIntyre, Penny McIntyre, Sally MacLellan, Vera Mather, Greg Matthews, Debbie Okun Hill, the pharmacy staff at Shoppers Drug Mart at Kent Street in Charlottetown, Dorothy Robichaud, Mary Sanderson, John and Mary Shattell, Kira Vermond, John Watson, Reita Watson, Nancy White, and Tipsy.